The
BODY BY SCIENCE
QUESTION AND ANSWER
BOOK

By Doug McGuff, MD and John Little

THE BODY BY SCIENCE
QUESTION AND ANSWER BOOK

TABLE OF CONTENTS

INTRODUCTION

"In all affairs it's a healthy thing now and then to hang a question mark on the things you have long taken for granted."
-- Bertrand Russell

As our readers might have anticipated, *The Body By Science Question & Answer Book* evolved out of a demand for more information (some of it general and some of it technical) from those trainees who wish to learn more about our evidence-based approach to exercise.

Our web site (www.bodybyscience.net) has filled this need to a large extent, but certain training (and most certainly rehabilitation) issues require more detailed explanation than a blog can often provide. *The Body By Science Question & Answer Book* addresses these questions and concerns and also allows for elaboration on certain key points that we presented in *Body By Science*.

Unlike *Body By Science*, however, this book assumes a certain level of understanding of the fundamental aspects of health and fitness on the part of the reader, and, thus, *Body By Science* should still be viewed as the reader's primary source of fundamental information on these topics. In this respect, the authors would consider this work to be a companion volume to *Body By Science*, rather than as something separate from it.

This book is broken into seven separate though interrelated sections, allowing the reader to go to whatever topic or section that is of most concern to him or her.

The breakdown is as follows:

Part One: Health & Fitness
In this section we examine and elaborate on how proper strength training contributes to the total health and fitness (not that these two concepts are co-joined) of the human organism. Topics such as layoffs from training, VO_2 Max testing, cardiovascular health, and other (for the moment more popular) approaches to it are examined and contrasted with resistance exercise.

Part Two: Bodybuilding

In this section we examine what is *really* required (as against what is popularly assumed) for human beings to make their bodies bigger and stronger. We also revisit the genetics issue and offer some insights that we have found through training our own clients on a one-on-one basis that have proven helpful in building muscle when other approaches have failed.

Part Three: Special Needs

In this section we take an in-depth look at how the trainee can deal with issues ranging from pregnancy to the common cold, in addition to presenting our approach to rehabilitating a host of ailments ranging from lower back pain to tendonitis.

Part Four: Training

In this section we answer questions about all aspects of training. Once the workout starts – and even after its finished – the trainee encounters many new experiences, from shaky limbs to post workout soreness (and many more besides). These issues are all addressed in this section of the book.

Part Five: Nutrition

In this section we examine what a healthy diet for humans truly consists of and also go into some depth on the role of insulin in the big picture of human health.

Part Six: Athletics

In this section we examine the concept of whether or not athletics – as a "conditioning" activity – is a safe option, and how to proceed with one's athletic endeavors in a manner that will augment (rather than hinder) one's performance. In addition, we scrutinize some of the coaching folklore that has endured (needlessly) in the athletic world.

Part Seven: Safety

In this section of the book we look at your exercise program with an eye toward keeping it safe over the long term. Issues such as breathing, gripping, exercise-induced headache, and recovery are covered (among many others).

The reader should know by now that it is our belief that proper strength training is something that every human being should do in order to maximize their functional ability and to live as healthy a life as possible. Hopefully this book will provide the reader with additional reasons and intellectual ammunition as to why this is so.

-- Doug McGuff, MD & John Little

PART ONE:
HEALTH AND FITNESS

HELPING THE PROCESS

QUESTION: *Apart from some of the information you have already provided, what can I do to maximize my workouts?*

ANSWER: There are several things you can do to maximize your workouts. The first is to understand why you're doing what you're doing and be ready to work *hard*. Remember that your body instinctively hates the inroading process and only by thoroughly understanding what your actual purpose is in working out, and maintaining your mental focus will you be able to inroad your muscles thoroughly, and thereby stimulate your body to produce the adaptive response you desire. Another thing that you can do (and that is imperative to your success) is to make sure that you really train to muscular failure, which is a process that simply takes time and practice. Most people mistake the sensation of discomfort, or a slowing down in contraction speed and the first mild burning sensation of lactic acid, for failure. This sensation is somewhat foreign to most people and can therefore lead to anxiety for some. Consequently, it is at this point that most subjects terminate their exercise. Instead, one must learn to live in this zone of unpleasantness for as long as one can; i.e., really dig deep. Many repetitions may require 20-seconds just to complete. And it's completely natural that when failure is truly reached you will not be calm; you will be desperately attempting to move the weight as the weight forces you into the negative phase of the last repetition. However, it is important that you realize that this is nothing to be panicky about, but rather a natural part of the process of deep muscular fatigue. Another thing you can do is to fight the temptation to unload the weight from your muscles by pushing quicker and then resting briefly and then pushing quickly again. Don't do this, however, as during the brief respite before each jab attempt, you are actually unloading the muscle (or muscles), which delays the inroading process and allows you to regain some of your strength, thus taking you farther away from inroad. And, finally, really make an effort to understand your objective and purpose for working out. The *assumed* objective of exercise for most people is to lift a heavier weight for a longer period of time or for more repetitions than they did the last time they worked out. The *real* objective, however, is to contract against the weight in a fashion that produces a maximum inroad or weakening of the muscles you are training, regardless of what ends up on your record sheet. For example, having your muscles contract against 180-pounds for a Time Under Load of 120-seconds that involved Valsalva, jabbing and resting in the lock out position of a leg press exercise, doesn't produce half of the inroad of a perfect set with 120-pounds performed for a Time Under Load of 95-seconds. Try to perform your repetitions in a manner that produces the most inroad and let your instructor (assuming you have one) worry about everything else.

STRENGTH REGAINED QUICKLY AFTER LAYOFFS

QUESTION: Is it possible to regain strength that was previously held after a lengthy layoff?

ANSWER: Absolutely. At Nautilus North we've had people that have taken up to four months off and come back to training stronger than they were prior to leaving. One of John Little's phone clients is a personal trainer that related that he had a client take a year off from training and come back stronger. In checking the science literature we note a study [1] in which subjects were trained for a period of 20 weeks, followed by 30 weeks of no training at all. The subjects then resumed training for another six weeks and quickly gained back the strength they had at the end of their initial 20 weeks of training. So, yes, it is not only possible, but realistically attainable to regain your strength even after a very sustained period of no training whatsoever.

RECONSIDERING WALKING FOR FAT LOSS

QUESTION: *I have always been told that walking is an activity that burns fat calories almost exclusively and therefore if one wants to lose body fat, one should walk or perform other aerobic activities as often as possible. You don't seem to buy into this notion. Why?*

ANSWER: We don't buy into the idea that daily cardio sessions are a must in order to lose body fat simply because such activity is not a particularly efficient means of doing so. Yes, such activities will burn *some* calories and, if calorie intake is closely regulated, they can contribute to losing body fat – but such activities are really such an ineffective way to burn calories that they're not really worth it. Don't misunderstand us; we do believe that it is important that one remain active (as this sends the appropriate metabolic message that carrying stored body fat is not only unnecessary, but has a negative effect), however it isn't necessary to have a regimented daily walking session performed at a modest level of intensity for this to happen. All that is required is that one be *normally* active. Apart from your high-intensity training workouts, we're not suggesting that one is best served by retreating into a foxhole and remaining motionless during the interval in between workouts, but we also don't advocate the other extreme that one should have to go out and walk or jog two miles every day. One must keep in mind that every time one outputs energy– however low the intensity – one is going to trigger a very strong biological prompt to put it back in. And if one outputs energy on a daily basis that is at a level that is higher than normal, it's going to take a will of iron to resist those constant biological prompts entreating you to input more energy into the system. This is why the sales of "cardio" machines, such as treadmills, have never been higher, and yet national levels of obesity have also never been higher. We had a client who went on a Breast Cancer walk – to raise money to fight breast cancer. She had previously been on the Nautilus North Fat Loss program (in which she worked out only once a week on two to three exercises and followed a well-balanced but calorie-reduced diet) and had lost over 20 pounds of body fat. However, she was in a hurry to lose even more body fat and the lure of "doing more" to accomplish this got the best of her. She saw this walk-a-thon as not only a great cause, but also a great opportunity to boost her activity levels (as she would have to walk 20 kilometers or so per session in preparing to do the big walk, which was 60 kilometers). And so she did – and at the end of that two-month period of doing no high-intensity training but lots of daily walking, she tested her body composition in the Bod Pod and was stunned to learn that she had actually gained six pounds of body fat for her efforts. And if you view what she experienced in the light of a hunter-gatherer background, you can readily understand the biologic message she was sending to her body by being in a calorie deficit and walking so much. From her body's vantage point she was an organism that was unable to find food and the incessant walking sent a message that she was perpetually unsuccessful in her hunting and gathering attempts. This caused her body to react as if it were in a starvation situation, which resulted in it issuing a command to store more energy (bodyfat) and downsize lean tissue, thus, reducing its daily metabolic rate.

KIDNEY FUNCTION AND RECOVERY

QUESTION: I read from a high-intensity author that overtraining is a result of producing metabolic waste products that the kidneys can't process quickly enough. He says that since the kidneys don't get any bigger as a result of exercise, but the work they are required to do increases as one gets stronger, that this is the reason why we have to spread out our training to once a week or less often.

ANSWER: While the general thought is intriguing, the reasoning – from a medical perspective – is flawed for the simple fact that you *can* greatly ramp up and ramp down glomerular filtration rate (GFR) based on demand. For example, if you develop a kidney stone in your right kidney, the glomerular filtration on that side will almost completely shut down and the glomerular filtration on the left side will more than double in order to compensate for it. If a friend of yours has renal failure and is on dialysis and wants a kidney transplant, if you want to donate one of your kidneys you can, and the other one can compensate for it without much difficulty at all. There are other factors at play that are responsible for our requiring a week or more to recover from intense exercise, rather than our glomerular filtration rate.

ADDITIONAL RECOVERY ISSUES

QUESTION: *I'm training once a week but my progress has stalled ever since I started a new job that requires shift work. I had started out so strong, going up in everything every time I went to the gym and now I'm not making any progress at all. I'm still training intensely and resting for a week, do you think I've tapped out my genetic potential after only four months?*

ANSWER: One thing we've learned over years of training and keeping records on clients on a one-on-one basis is that if a certain client is less responsive you've got to look at the *total context* of what is going on in his or her life. It has been our experience that clients who live significantly stressful lifestyles are the ones who may require even *more* recovery time in between their workouts. For instance, one of Doug's clients is a fellow ER physician who worked the night shift full time and had four children that required his attention during the day. And what Doug found was that his physician friend could not make any improvements in strength unless he took even more time off in between workouts. So the trainers at Ultimate Exercise (Doug's facility) kept extending the Doctor's "off" days until they found that, reliably, a training frequency of once every twelve days worked best for him. If he attempted to train on the tenth or the eleventh day after his previous workout, he would never register any improvement. With a proper approach to training, which is inclusive of proper record keeping, this type of optimal training frequency is detectable and with the *Body By Science* approach to training we can actually produce results in people when no other training approach can. And the reason for this is that we're not afraid to figure out exactly how long it takes people to recover and produce an adaptation to the exercise stimulus. And for poor responders this can be a very long time. In some of our less responsive clients we've found that a *minimum* of 12 days needs to elapse between workouts before they show improvement. Without having this time off not only would they not make any progress, but they would actually regress. And as with the client example cited above, this is particularly true for people that are average or poor responders and that also have stressful lifestyles (i.e., rotating shift work, small children that require constant attention, economic or employment stress, etc.). Anything that produces a significant stress or disruption of one's sleep cycles will result in one having to train with less volume and less frequency in order to produce optimal results. It should be pointed out that adaptive energy is not something that is just dedicated to recovering from workouts; it's dedicated to one's whole life. Someone that is embroiled in a lawsuit, or going through a divorce, or taking care of an ill parent, or starting a new job -- all of these things will delay one's recovery ability as they are things that make demands upon one's limited reserve of adaptive energy.

THE GENESIS OF GLOBAL METABOLIC CONDITIONING

QUESTION: *I'm fascinated by your concept of Global Metabolic Conditioning because it makes such sense! Why would anyone want to settle for only one segment (such as the aerobic component) of the totality of metabolic health? I'm curious, however, as to how you came up with the concept of Global Metabolic Conditioning?*

ANSWER: The concept of Global Metabolic Conditioning is entirely the achievement of Dr. Doug McGuff. Consequently, it would be best if your question were answered directly by him:

It struck me – as it does everybody else – that when you perform high-intensity exercise, you are experiencing something that is *completely* different from any form of exertion that you've ever done. That subjective experience of actually going through that kind of workout and feeling the difference, and feeling what your capabilities become after performing that kind of exercise, is unbelievable. You realize as an immediate consequence that you are training things here that nothing else can. So what is it that's going on that's different here? Because you can run, jog, cycle, swim – whatever – but until someone has taken you through a four or five set workout that's high-intensity and takes only 12-minutes -- but after that 12-minutes has elapsed you realize that this is completely different than anything you've ever experienced! There's nothing else that holds a candle to this! That is what triggered my thought that there are other metabolic things going on here than is popularly thought about. But what is that something else? When I went back home after one of my high-intensity workouts I went to my old med school bookstore and went through the bio-chemistry section, hoping that I would find something that would help me with this nagging sensation of what was so different about this experience compared to anything else I had done. It was then that I came across the textbook *Biochemistry At A Glance,* And the premise of this textbook was, "Let's look at metabolism as a road map." On the inside cover of the textbook and in the introductory chapter they showed a bird's eye view of a road map of London that displayed all the roads and the pathways and streets and how you get from one place to the other. And it talked about how taxi drivers in London have to study this map and learn it. And how having an aerial view of it all lets you see how everything ties together and where the best routes are and that sort of thing. And what they did was take this concept of an aerial view and apply it to a cell and then they illustrated in a street map form all of the metabolic pathways. And once I was able to get that aerial view, so to speak, of all the metabolic pathways and how they link together, that's when I said, "Okay, what's happening here is we're now working hard enough where we have to tap every metabolic pathway maximally, whereas other forms of exertion don't do that. But when you bring a demand to the organism of such a magnitude that it has to use *every* metabolic resource possible to meet the demands of that exertion, this produces an involvement of all aspects of metabolism at a much higher level, which is how I came to the conclusion that this is a "global metabolic conditioning" that's taking place. It is not an *isolated* metabolic conditioning; it's not a conditioning that is trying to place an emphasis only one particular metabolic pathway. We're looking at the whole cell from above realizing that this entire cell connects to the cardiovascular system, and not just, say, the aerobic sub-segment of metabolism. So when you do exercise like what I've experienced that seems so different, it's different because we're performing a global metabolic conditioning and not an isolated metabolic conditioning.

-- Doug McGuff, MD

HIT AND CARDIO

QUESTION: If I perform strength training along the lines of what you advocate in Body By Science, *how will this improve my cardiovascular system?*

ANSWER: To understand this better, you need to look at the picture of a cell that we illustrated on page 23 of *Body By Science.* Note that the cell has a liquid portion, which is the cytoplasm, and this is where all the glycolytic/anaerobic enzymes exist. Note also that it has mitochondria, and it is here where all of aerobic metabolism occurs. But when you look at that picture of the entire cell, you've got to ask yourself, "Is this entire cell connected to the cardiovascular system or by what means of magic is *only* the mitochondria connected to the heart and blood vessels?" There has been such a long culture created by Ken Cooper and the aerobics craze that now people believe that the aerobic subsystem of metabolism somehow bypasses all other metabolic components to link *directly* to cardiovascular health, when, in fact, that is just a specific metabolic adaptation of that entire cell. In other words, the entire cell is served by the cardiovascular system. Moreover, one can make other specific metabolic adaptations that involve that entire cell that are not aerobic but that will also be addressed by the cardiovascular system. In other words, all of these metabolic adaptations that we think are cardiovascular are not; i.e., there is no central cardiovascular adaptation, per se, taking place. The reason that one can observe measurable changes in cardiovascular parameters is because of specific metabolic adaptations that occur in the periphery in the muscle itself. The VO_2 Max test, for example, measures oxygen uptake, and therefore if aerobic capacity is really a central cardiovascular adaptation, we ought to be able to tell or measure this. And in *Body By Science* we reported of a very simple yet elegant study wherein they had subjects train to enhance their VO_2 Max through steady-state activity involving just their right arm and right leg. And the subjects did show a percentage increase in their VO_2 Max – when they tested the right arm and right leg. However, when they tested their left arm and left leg, there was no evident improvement in their VO_2 Max. And when the experimenters tested both the right arm and right leg and the left arm and left leg simultaneously there was an improvement in VO_2 Max that was just 50% of what it was when they only tested the right arm and right leg. So when people talk about these adaptations that are popularly referred to as "cardiovascular," they are actually referring to adaptations that are going on in muscle tissue. It is muscle that is the window to the body, and the degree to which you have improved your level of muscle mass is the degree to which you positively effect all markers of health. Not only your cardiovascular health but health markers that we don't typically consider, such as gastrointestinal transit time (as the weights of many different organs in the body will be in some degree proportional to one's muscle mass, and as a consequence, their functioning is going to be directly proportional to the functional ability of one's muscles). So the degree to which we can strengthen and add muscle tissue to a given individual will be the degree to which we can increase the functional capacity throughout his or her body. So the idea that you have to perform some form of activity that attempts, in a false sense of what's possible, to isolate a particular subsegment of metabolism because we think it will benefit the cardiovascular system is folly, because the cardiovascular system just does not work that way. And, indeed, if one looks at the way that the metabolic subsystems of the body actually function one will see that if one really wants to maximally stimulate one's aerobic pathway one can only do so by maximizing one's level of anaerobic metabolism. Because the glyolytic process (whereby glucose is converted to pyruvate) can cycle much faster than the aerobic process in the mitochondria can process it, the glycolytic process can produce pyruvate at a rate much faster than the mitcchondria can use it. So performing *anaerobic* exercise is the only way in which one can be certain that one has maximally stimulated one's aerobic system and caused it to cycle as fast as it can possibly go. Moreover, pyruvate is processed out of the body through the aerobic system at a slow and steady pace, so when one finishes one's high-intensity workout, the lactic acid that was produced by the anaerobic exercise is converted back into pyruvate for metabolization through the aerobic cycle. What this means in practical terms is that you can be sitting around after your workout, perhaps doing something productive like writing a book or studying for your PhD, and while you're doing that you're actually getting the equivalent aerobic workout of steady-state activity – during the "recovery" period after high-intensity exercise as the lactic acid that you stock piled gets converted to pyruvate and processed through your aerobic system. So the perceived health benefit that many people think *only* steady-state activity can provide, actually occurs in the recovery period after high-intensity training. And the big advantage high-intensity training has over more conventional "aerobic" training is that the former actually addresses your musculature and does something to maximize its functional capability (which really does have a more direct effect on health parameters).

THE McMASTER STUDIES

QUESTION: The two studies conducted by McMaster University that you cited in Body By Science *are fascinating! What do you think was the biggest thing that you learned from them?*

ANSWER: For over four decades it was believed that you had to perform a steady-state activity for a minimum of 20-minutes in order to thoroughly engage the aerobic system. And that seemed to be turned on its head experimentally when studies conducted at McMaster University revealed that a doubling of aerobic capacity could be achieved by a grand total of six-minutes of exercise a week. The subjects didn't have to engage in their "cardio" session for a minimum of 20-minutes straight, instead they worked their muscles vigorously for 30-seconds and then took a four-minute rest, and repeated this three more times. This belief that "you have to be in your target heart range for "X" amount of time to get any cardiovascular benefit" was shown to be completely arbitrary. And this assumption was based on the fact that the level of metabolic adaptation that occurs with the performance of low-intensity exercise is so minimal that the volume and frequency of it must be increased dramatically to obtain any effect from it at all as, on its own, it certainly wasn't a potent enough stimulus for the adaptation to persist. Consequently, a neurotic type of mentality arose of, "you have to do *more* of it" – and you did because it was a very minimal metabolic adaptation brought by a minimal stimulus/intensity, with the result that it deconstructed quite quickly as there wasn't a demanding enough impetus or reason for the body to preserve it. However, if you pursue that same metabolic adaptation for your aerobic system via a means of high-intensity muscular work, it takes very little of this type of stimulus for the adaptation to occur and to be well preserved. The lead researcher of the McMaster study, Professor Martin Gibala, told one of the authors that he believed that the researchers probably could have produced the same results with even less exercise than (a total of) 6-minutes a week. Interestingly, in his newspaper interviews,

Professor Gibala was almost apologetic for establishing clinically that there was a more efficient way to stimulate the cardiovascular system! Many exercise scientists have a fear of turning over the applecart with new discoveries, when they should be delighted and proud of their achievement. A more appropriate approach would have been, "We've found the answer -- let's see where it takes us!" Why not press on to see exactly how *little* exercise is required to maximally stimulate the aerobic system? That aside, the McMaster Studies put the lie to the belief that one had to workout at least three times a week for a minimum of 20-minutes a workout in order to get "cardio." In fact, it reduced this number by almost two-thirds! And if performing four or five 30-second intervals are all that's required, that could just as well be achieved – from the standpoint of both your muscles and cardiovascular system – by working your muscles intensely with four or five different exercises, such as a "Big 5" routine consisting of a Leg Press, a Compound Row, A Chest Press, a Pulldown and an Overhead Press. So the McMaster studies made a very strong case for short, intense workout sessions (as little as two-minutes of total training time per workout) stimulating profound improvements in one's aerobic capacity.

HIGH-INTENSITY TRAINING BENEFITS FOR ENDURANCE ATHLETES

QUESTION: My wife and I are tandem cyclists and, as an MD, I appreciate your scientific approach very much. However, I'm curious as to how you would explain the fact that runners, cyclists and other "endurance athletes" get faster with current training programs such as those that emphasize interval training?

ANSWER: The reason is simply because interval programs are of higher intensity than their steady-state counterpart. Also, the degree of improvement one can obtain from endurance exercise (i.e., low-intensity steady state exercise) is achieved relatively quickly and easily, and additional volume on top of that does not result in additional metabolic adaptations from exercise at that intensity level. In other words, someone can train to run a marathon by performing steady-state activity of much shorter distances, but additional distance added on to that will not result in any further metabolic adaptations for that level of exertion. And what we're starting to see in endurance exercise protocols that involve training for marathons or other long distance events is that these athletes are now supplementing their lower intensity steady-state activity (necessary to train the aerobic metabolic pathway specifically for these types of events) with higher-intensity activity that then stimulates the body to produce adaptations beyond what is possible with the more conventional steady-state levels of exertion. And a lot of what makes and breaks athletes in terms of their performance in endurance competition are the periods of time during the event where they have to ramp up their level of exertion. And this can be because segments of the course that they're participating in are uphill and thus require a higher level of exertion, or there may be periods of time where in events such as cycling the athlete has to do a breakaway to try and distance himself from a group, and that requires the athlete to perform an all out sprint. In the case of cyclists, this might also be encountered when the cyclist has fallen off the pack and no longer has anyone to draft, which, again, will require a significantly higher degree of exertion. This is where the interval training that the athlete has performed at a higher level of intensity assumes relevance, as it is what has stimulated the necessary metabolic adaptations that allow the athlete to do these things successfully. In other words, if the athlete desires such higher order metabolic improvements, then he has to raise the intensity of the training stimulus, and the higher the stimulus/intensity he imposes on his musculature, the greater the improvements that his body is going to produce. Steady-state endurance athletes benefit from performing high-intensity training in many ways, one of which being that such training stimulates the accessibility of alternate metabolic pathways that the body can rely upon when the steady-state activity has been carried on for so long that the athlete taps out his glycogen stores, allowing the athlete to continue to perform at a high level after a period of high exertion has already transpired. When an athlete performs high-intensity training, he cultivates the ability to raise his lactate threshold by conditioning the Cori Cycle, which serves to take the lactate that is produced from high levels of muscular exertion and deliver it to the liver where it is recycled back into glucose. This process takes the blood buffer systems that maintain a normal pH during periods of lactic acidosis and allows them to produce higher levels of 2,3-bisphosphoglycerate (2,3-BPG) that allow for easier delivery of oxygen to the tissues. And all of these different metabolic adaptations are brought about through high-intensity exertion, and are very useful to an endurance athlete during those periods in the competition where he has to ramp up his energy output and also during situations where he has gone for so long that he is starting to run out of substrate and now must rely on other metabolic sources to fuel his on-going muscular contractions. This was established during the McMaster Study cited earlier, in which higher intensity interval work (consisting of four 30-second intervals with up to 4-minutes of rest in between) was shown to double the cardiovascular endurance of subjects compared to the control group.

LACTATE THRESHOLD TRAINING

QUESTION: What is really occurring when one performs a training program that emphasizes so-called "lactate threshold" training?

ANSWER: In actuality there are several things happening; first, one is working at a higher level of exertion, and thus producing a higher order of stimulus and the metabolic adaptations that occur as a result of one's producing a higher order of stimulus are more profound and better preserved by the body for longer periods of time. Second, one cultivates the metabolic ability to continue to perform muscular work of a metabolically demanding nature long after one has outstripped the capability of one's aerobic metabolism to continue to supply energy to the process. In other words, when one has tapped the aerobic subsystem for supplying energy, the glycolysis cycle is engaged to the full, with the result that it is producing pyruvate faster than the mitochondria within the aerobic pathways can use it. And when this happens one is operating at a level of intensity where the body must now cultivate alternative metabolic adaptations that will allow one to continue to produce effort after one has exceeded the aerobic system's capability of supplying energy. This results in an up-regulation of the metabolic systems that allow one to work hard after that point in time, and involves the up-regulation of the enzymatic systems involved in the Cori Cycle (the process whereby lactate is brought back to the liver and converted back into pyruvate so that it can undergo the process of gluconeogenesis to convert it into glucose that can then be used to serve as substrate for continued muscular exertion). Third, one will become far more efficient at blowing off carbon dioxide, which, in turn, serves to buffer one's blood pH. This process allows one to produce more of the protein components of blood that allow one to buffer against lactic acidosis, which can often rise to such high levels that it interferes with the muscles ability to continue to contract. Consequently, under extreme conditions one is going to be stimulating all of the metabolic systems that serve to augment the aerobic system, thus allowing the muscles to continue in their task of contracting for longer periods of time. The body accomplishes this by increasing its production of Erthyropoetin, which results in one's having a little higher content of red blood cells to assist in the transport of oxygen. In addition, one's body is going to start to enhance the metabolism of 2,3-disphosphoglycerate, which is a molecule that the body produces that actually serves to alter the shape of the hemoglobin molecule making it bind oxygen less aggressively. When one first hears this it, admittedly, sounds like it would be a process that one wouldn't want to happen, but it should be pointed out that a hemoglobin molecule is a very aggressive allosteric binder of oxygen, which means that if one molecule of oxygen is bound, it actually changes its shape so that it will attract oxygen even more. And then a second molecule will cause it to change shape again, so that it attracts even more oxygen molecules, which is followed by a third, and fourth molecule, which serves to extend the process even further, so that by the time one has bound four molecules of oxygen on the hemoglobin, it's so tightly bound that it's reluctant to give it up. So oxygen delivery to the various systems of the body is actually predicated on hemoglobin binding oxygen molecules less tightly. And that's what 2,3-disphosphoglycerate does; it binds to the hemoglobin molecule, affecting its shape in such a way that it releases oxygen more easily, so that as blood circulates to tissues that are now shifting to a more anaerobic metabolism, one will actually increase one's 2,3-disphosphoglycerate, which, then, affects the shape of the hemoglobin molecule so that it releases oxygen more easily into the system. So anaerobic lactate-threshold training actually enhances one's aerobic capacity because one's body is able to develop these profound metabolic adaptations that then serve to allow one's aerobic subsystem to continue to contribute at a high level for longer periods of time.

MORE ON VO$_2$ MAX

QUESTION: In the textbook Essentials of Exercise Physiology (chapter 8, Evaluating Energy Generating Capacities During Exercise) it is stated that, "In essence, VO$_2$ Max represents a fundamental measure in exercise physiology and serves as a standard to compare performance estimates of aerobic capacity and endurance fitness." Also, on the same page, it is stated that, "a leveling off or peaking over in oxygen uptake during increasing exercise intensity signifies attainment of maximum capacity to aerobic metabolism; i.e., a true VO$_2$ Max." How, then, would you explain this peaking over in oxygen uptake, which is actually a reduction in VO$_2$ Max with all-out efforts, and increasing grades in speed on the treadmill?

ANSWER: This is a huge assumption based upon multiple assumptions. One of the assumptions is that the VO$_2$ Max test is equally accurate at all levels of exertion. It must be remembered that the maximum oxygen uptake test was originally designed to measure oxygen utilization and metabolism of subjects at *rest*. And in order to get a measurement of oxygen uptake one has to have a closed system that measures oxygen consumption and expired CO_2. In other words what is required is a machine that can measure all of the inspired oxygen and the expired CO_2 and then perform a measurement of the oxygen in inspired air versus the oxygen in expired air in order to make the necessary calculations – and this is predicated on equipment that is performing this calculation in a closed system with a very tightly fitting mask and a level of dead space of air that is known and calculated for. The dead space in this instance would be the tubing that runs between the mask and the equipment that is delivering the oxygen and measuring the difference between the two. And that's a measurement that has proven to be very accurate at low levels of exertion or when the subject is at rest. However, when the level of exertion is raised to higher levels, particularly when the subject does so on a treadmill or ergometer, that subject will be bobbing and jerking up and down with the result that any possibility of maintaining a tight seal of the mask is compromised. Another assumption is that other metabolic factors aren't coming into play that the test simply isn't engineered to take into account owing to the fact that it only measures (albeit imperfectly) oxygen utilization. Factors touched on in the answer to the previous question such as blood buffer systems, 2,3-disphosphoglycerate, and other metabolic factors all contribute to the process and cannot be isolated out of the total picture as they are all engaged simultaneously. Another assumption is that the "dead space" of the tubing isn't changing continuously, when in fact it is. Consequently, during the VO_2 Max text, what had been assumed to be a known and fixed volume of gas in a fixed tube running from the subject to the machinery, the volume of the tubing is changing with each bump and jostle of the subject. Consequently, when a subject is using his muscles at a high level of exertion, the leveling off that is detected by the VO_2 Max test may in fact be due to the inherent inaccuracy of the equipment under these conditions. Consequently, loose fitting seals, volume quantities that are imperfectly known, and the fact that the aerobic system has maximally contributed and other subsystems of metabolism are now contributing to the ongoing exertion can all lead to faulty assumptions regarding why a leveling off or peaking over in oxygen uptake can occur during an increased intensity in exercise. But the real fatal flaw with VO_2 ^{Max} testing is confusing this drop or leveling off in oxygen consumption with a leveling off of cardiovascular function at that level of exertion, as these two factors definitely do *not* directly correlate. As we've indicated, one's cardiovascular system can continue to function for a period of time at very high levels beyond this leveling off period owing to the involvement of the other substrate systems. The current concept of the "leveling off" factor is predicated on the notion that there is some *central* cardiovascular component that is limiting oxygen delivery to the working muscles. The assumption being that VO_2 ^{Max} tracks on a perfect one-to-one ratio with cardiac output factors, such that when one witnesses the VO_2 ^{Max} leveling off it is because cardiovascular capabilities have leveled off, and, therefore, one is unable to deliver any additional oxygen to one's working muscles. That is the typical or more popular notion in exercise physiology as to why this leveling off effect occurs but we do not believe that such is the case, but rather that the leveling off that is seen may be more a component of the test itself, as opposed to something tangible that is actually being measured. There is support for our position in the scientific literature, particularly in the work of a physiologist/researcher by the name of Timothy Noakes from South Africa. In an article that presented a snapshot of Noakes' views, the author stated:

The traditional view of VO_2 ^{Max} owes a great deal to the work of A.V. Hill who conducted experiments on exercising men in Manchester, England in the 1920s. Hill and colleagues proposed that there's an upper limit to oxygen uptake (VO_2 ^{Max}), that there are inner individual differences in this variable and that VO_2 ^{Max} is limited by the circulatory and/or respiratory systems. They demonstrated that oxygen uptake increases linearly with running speed, but in some subjects it eventually "reaches a maximum beyond which no effort can drive it," a phenomenon now referred to as the VO_2 plateau. In recent years, Timothy Noakes has strongly criticized Hill's concept of VO_2 ^{Max}. He maintains that the absence of a VO_2 ^{Max} plateau in some subjects is proof that oxygen delivery is not a limiting factor for VO_2 ^{Max}. This view fails to recognize that the plateau is not the principle evidence for a cardio-respiratory limitation. Noakes rejects the VO_2 ^{Max} paradigm of A.V. Hill in its entirety. The alternative paradigm that he proposes is that endurance performance is limited by muscle factors. Noakes suggests that the best distance runners have muscle characteristics that allow them to achieve their higher running speeds, and since running speed is linearly related to oxygen uptake, an indirect consequence of this is that they will have higher VO_2 ^{Max} values. This is exactly the opposite of how the relationship of VO_2 ^{Max} and running speed at the end of a maximal exercise test should be viewed. [2]

Another study that was cited in *Body By Science* [3] is worth reconsidering here as it measured VO_2 ^{Max} in subjects and then trained them for improvement in VO_2 ^{Max} using just their right arms and right legs on an ergometer. After the training period the subjects VO_2 ^{Max} was retested using the right arm and the right leg together, and revealed a certain percentage improvement in the subjects' VO_2 ^{Max}. But when they tested the untrained left arm and left leg the experimenters discovered that there were no improvements at all in their VO_2 ^{Max}. Therefore, the assumption that improvements in VO_2 ^{Max} indicated central improvements in the cardio-respiratory system was found to be without merit. The experimenters further discovered that if both the trained and untrained limbs were tested together there was an improvement in VO_2 ^{Max} of roughly 50 percent, indicating that all of the measured improvements in VO_2 ^{Max} occurred because of changes in the periphery of the trained *muscles*. The results of this study strongly support Noakes' contention regarding the inefficiency of VO_2 ^{Max} testing. According to Noakes:

A popular concept in the exercise theories holds that fatigue develops during exercise of moderate to high intensity when the capacity of the cardio-respiratory system to provide oxygen to the exercising muscles falls behind their demand, inducing anaerobic metabolism. But this cardiovascular/anaerobic model is unsatisfactory because, one, a more rigorous analysis indicates that the first organ to be effected by anaerobiosis during maximal exercise would likely be the heart, not the skeletal muscles. This probability was fully appreciated by the pioneering exercise physiologists A.V. Hill, A. Brock and D.B. Dill, but has been systematically ignored by modern exercise physiologists. Two, no study has yet definitely established the presence of either anaerobiosis, hypoxia or eschemia of skeletal muscle during maximal exercise. And three, the model is unable to explain why exercise terminates in a variety of conditions including prolonged exercise, exercise in the heat and at altitude and in those with chronic diseases of the heart and lungs without any evidence for skeletal muscle anaerobiosis, hypoxia or eschemia and before there is full activation of the total skeletal muscle mass. And four, cardiovascular and other measurements believed to relate to skeletal muscle anaerobiosis include the maximum oxygen uptake consumption ($VO_2{}^{Max}$) and the anaerobic threshold, are indifferent predictors of exercise capacity in athletes of similar abilities. This review considers four additional models that need to be considered when factors limiting either short duration, maximal, or prolonged sub-maximal exercise are evaluated. The additional models are:

1.) The energy supply/energy depletion model
2.) The muscle power/muscle recruitment model
3.) The biomechanical model
4.) The psychological model

By reviewing the features of these models, the review provides a broad overview of physiological, metabolic and biomechanical factors that may limit exercise performance under different exercise conditions. A more complete understanding of fatigue during exercise and the relevance of the adaptations that develop with training requires that the potential relevance of each model to fatigue under different conditions with exercise must be considered. [4]

In other words, the fall off that the physiologists are seeing occurs because of metabolic adaptive factors that are occurring within the muscle, and not because of something that's occurring in the central cardiovascular system. And this is where high-intensity resistance training comes to the fore. When one looks at Noakes' "energy supply/energy depletion model" one immediately sees the importance of the role of muscle mass, as these are the storehouses of glycogen, and, thus, the means of supplying glucose to the demanding system for longer periods of time. Noakes' "muscle power/muscle recruitment model" refers to the fact that if one is stronger, the performance of a given level of work requires the recruitment of a smaller number of fibers and, therefore, the metabolic support of the mechanical functioning of fewer fibers. Consequently, this may give the appearance of an improved VO_2^{Max}. The "biomechanical model" refers to the fact that the mechanics of a particular activity become more efficient over time, which is why if one trains to improve one's VO_2^{Max} on a treadmill but is tested on a bicycle ergometer, one won't manifest any evidence of that improvement (or at least it won't be as much as one would expect), owing to the fact that most of the improvements that one witnesses will simply be improvements in economy of motion and mechanical efficiency. And finally the "psychological model" Noakes refers to is his belief that there is a central nervous system governor that inhibits motor unit recruitment (and motor unit recruitment at higher levels) as a means of protecting the heart from anaerobic metabolism. As myocardial ischemia is very dangerous and life threatening, Noakes believes that there's an internal governor that creates this plateau through muscular effects, rather than central cardiovascular effects. And that also accounts for a plateau of VO_2^{Max} [1] The VO_2^{Max} test, then, has serious limitations and the assumptions about the test are largely incorrect. While some physiologists believe that the test is a measure of central cardiovascular capacity and, thus, that improvements represent improvements in one's central cardiovascular symptoms, that very elegantly performed and simple study on VO_2^{Max} that we cited in *Body By Science*, combined with Noakes' pioneering research has caused many to question the validity of that belief.

PALEO FITNESS

QUESTION: I'm intrigued by Body By Science *and how you base a lot of your fitness recommendations on our Hunter/Gatherer heritage. However, I note that another Doctor (Dr. Boyd Eaton), along with Melvin Konner and Anthropology Assistant Professor Marjorie Shostak, in their book* The Paleontolithic Prescription, *share many of your views about Hunter/Gatherers influencing our present genome. However, on the matter of fitness they state:*

> ...there should be a relationship between endurance exercise and longevity. To "prove" conclusively such a relationship is statistically difficult, but mounting evidence tends to confirm its existence. Dr. Ralph Paffenbarger has tracked the health and life-styles of nearly 17,000 Harvard College alumni. His data strongly indicate that, in this group at least, regular physical activity extends length of life, chiefly because it decreases the risk of cardiovascular mortality. Those alumni whose habitual activity levels required expenditures of at least 2,000 calories per week had 50 percent less risk of heart attack than did their less-energetic classmates. Paffenbarger's figures suggest that each hour of strenuous exercise – jogging, vigorous walking, bicycling, single's tennis, and so on – adds one to three hours of increased life expectancy. In other words, people who remain physically active and fit can add up to two years of life by this means alone. For the Harvard alumni this was true regardless of age and was independent of other risk factors such as smoking, hypertension, and obesity. [5]

What say you to this counter view of exercise and longevity?

ANSWER: When you cited the quote, "Paffenbarger's figures suggest that each hour of strenuous exercise – jogging, vigorous walking, bicycling, single's tennis, and so on – adds one to three hours of increased life expectancy," our first response was, "How did he make THAT calculation?" Don't forget that on page 193 of that same book the authors report another study of

Paffenbarger's that involved longshoremen in San Francisco, which the authors summarized as follows:

"Those who performed *heavy physical labor* [our italics] had lower mortality rates from heart disease than did workers whose jobs were less physically demanding. The work pattern for the longshoremen – which involved repeated *bursts of peak effort rather than continuous, lower-level energy output* – was *more comparable to strength training than it was to aerobic exercise.*"

The association between *some* muscular work and longevity may be linked in causation, but if you were to analyze it on a deeper level, you would find that the benefit (longevity in this case) was attributable to very brief periods of time where the people who were studied had exertion levels that were actually of fairly high-intensity. So the hard intense muscular work that the longshoreman performed during a brief three-to-five-minute period in his six hour day may have been responsible for all of the risk reduction markers and everything else of benefit. And so it goes with all forms of physical activity. For instance, the jogger that's out jogging five days a week may encounter one hill on his route where his muscles really have to work at a high-intensity level as he surmounts it. This would really tap into his glycogen stores and, thus, provide the major benefit he experienced from his jogging for that day. There might be something condensed within that entire context that might be accounting for the reported association between activity and longevity. But just running on the assumption that activity, per se, explains the effect does not take this into account, nor does it consider the rather confounding variable that people who are intrinsically healthy tend to be more active. So it may actually be evidence of a reversal of cause and effect that they were looking at and then just making an assumption. Often times increased activity levels are simply an expression of the joy of being physiologically superior to your cohorts. But what we've found is that if we train people the way we do, we don't have to give them a regimented program of increasing their activities, as their activity levels will spontaneously rise. You may note that a dog that is dying of spleen cancer will not be active, but rather will lie around and moan. However, when that condition isn't present a dog will typically be observed running around, getting into garbage, barking at people walking by, etc. In other words, the healthier the animal (including the human animal), the more active the animal. And if positive changes take place in one's global metabolic conditioning, then just like the healthy dog, one's activity level will spontaneously increase. We've seen it over and over again: a stronger person can do more and will do more because it requires less energy from them to do so when they are stronger than it did when they were weaker.

A FINAL THOUGHT

QUESTION: *So many people have it in their minds that they still have to train many hours and days per week in order to get stronger and to improve their fitness levels – including their cardiovascular fitness. How can you get these people to change their minds about this?*

ANSWER: One, we'd like to point out that this notion has not always existed. There were very successful physical conditioning programs done in the early 20th century that brought great results to many people but that were later drowned out by louder more commercial voices. Second, the vast majority of people fall out of their exercise programs because they don't have the time for it; that is, they're being asked to engage in exercise too frequently, and, as a consequence, even if such an approach did produce outstanding results, the time cost is beyond the realm of affordability for most people. However, such programs – which are by far the most prevalent – are quite clearly not producing results; i.e., obesity is greater now than ever before and people are less fit than they were 50 years ago. It's little wonder that people are losing interest in exercise and dropping out. Indeed, the drop out rate in exercise programs is higher than any other human endeavor, and it is so for a reason – because we have been listening to the wrong people. When someone is standing up as an expert -- particularly someone with inordinate physical development -- and offering exercise advice, you need to ask yourself, "Do I *look* anything like this person?" And, "Am I listening to this person because of the way they *look*?" And if your answers to these questions are "no" and "yes," respectively, then you need to check your premises and start over. Because the real biology of the situation is that *it doesn't take much* properly performed exercise to stimulate a good adaptive result -- and the reason is because *we are an adaptive organism.* And, consequently, it isn't in the nature of things that we should have to invest a lot of time into a biological activity in order to reap good results if we have a history of survival as a highly evolved species (which we do). So think about it in those terms and the process and principles of what we are advocating will make a lot more sense to you. And also recognize that the current notions of exercise frequency are predicated upon a selection bias and commercial interests. The selection bias has occurred because there are people that have superior physiques and that express the joy of those superior physiques by high volumes of physical activity and then try to sell to us that such high volume activity was responsible for their physiques rather than the other way round.

Decades ago, Nautilus machine inventor Arthur Jones made gave us a parable about aliens coming down to our planet and going to a basketball game. Once at the game the aliens observed a species out on the basketball court bouncing an orange ball and all of them were seven-feet tall. And when they turned their many eyes to the stands they noted that the species that were sitting in the bleachers were all shorter and fatter than the species out on the court. And the aliens concluded through the process of simple observation that bouncing an orange ball made one species tall and lean, while sitting in a bleacher seat made another species short and fat. This is a parable that explains the selection bias we are talking about. But instead of aliens, we have ourselves, the vast majority of whom are truly aliens to the realm of exercise. And instead of seeing tall people bouncing basketballs, we are seeing people that are naturally muscular, lean and fit who are performing high levels of activity. And we have made the same false assumption that the aliens did; we are assuming that it is the type (and volume) of this activity that is responsible for producing the extraordinary physical attributes and capabilities these people display, when, in fact, it was their extraordinary physical attributes and capabilities that have allowed them to engage in such voluminous activity. Consequently, many people believe that they should be doing more activity – despite its proven history of doing damage and shortening lives in the vast majority of people who do not share the genetic gifts necessary to tolerate such prolonged bouts of physical activity without ill consequence. From a physiological standpoint, from a fitness standpoint, from a health standpoint and, yes, from an exercise standpoint, proper training performed once a week is all that most of the population can tolerate and all that they need to perform. However, as one gets stronger, one will notice something else happens– a simultaneous increase in one's activity levels. In other words, one will become more active as a direct result of the fact that one's physique is now stronger and better conditioned– it doesn't work the other way round. Because as one gets better conditioned as a result of the type of exercise that we advocate, one's activity levels will naturally rise as a simple expression of the enjoyment of one's improved physiology. And, perhaps most importantly, one will enjoy life far more fully, and with less wear and tear and greater functional ability than is possible by any other approach. And the price of these benefits is a mere 12-minutes once a week.

PART TWO:
BODYBUILDING

BUILDING BIGGER MUSCLES

QUESTION: I like your program very much and it makes perfect sense. However, I really want to build my muscles up to be as big as possible (like a bodybuilder). Will this program help me to gain maximum muscle mass?

ANSWER: An individual who comes to us wanting to build maximum muscle size would be put on the same program that we put everyone else on for two reasons; one, we believe that it's the best starting point to produce meaningful results. Two, it's an excellent starting point for accurately assessing an individual's potential for building muscle mass. It must be remembered that what a person *desires* may not necessarily be what they are *capable of achieving*. A lot of young men will come to a gym or a trainer with an aspiration of being a competitive bodybuilder (or at least looking like one). But wishing it and being able to do it are two completely separate things. And while it may be true that if someone has the required genetic potential to be a competitive bodybuilder that there might be some needs that our "Big 5" routine does not accommodate, and which will need to be accommodated in order for such a person to maximize his bodybuilding potential (as if one is in possession of that kind of genetic potential, it probably also means that one is in possession of certain genetic traits that effect one's tolerance of intensity, volume and frequency such that one's workout might need to be up-regulated at times), the fact remains that the "Big 5" is still the best place to start. The reason being that if an individual starts his training with a good, basic program, he will quickly uncover what he has in terms of potential for building massive muscles. And it's not going to be a result of one coincidentally having found a good match with a particular protocol so much as it will be a case of the fact that if someone has the potential to be a competitive bodybuilder it will be evident early on in one's training (and sometimes even before they've even seriously taken up any form of training) -- and it will be evidenced through working out on an extremely basic training program.

THE NORM AND THE EXCEPTION

QUESTION: I really want to gain about 30 pounds of muscle. I've been training the conventional way for about three years but haven't seen much in the way of gains after Year One. Will the Body By Science *program allow me to accomplish my goal?*

ANSWER: Not really – because your goal sounds to us to be unrealistic. If you've been training for three years and you believe you're still 30 pounds of muscle shy of your goal, then it's highly unlikely that you possess the genetics necessary to achieve such a goal. Moreover, after a year or so of training, even a gain of five pounds of pure muscle over the course of a year is a huge achievement. And if you break that down on a daily basis it's almost undetectable. The problem is in false expectations that are promulgated by the bodybuilding and fitness industry that promote images of genetic marvels that are a couple of standard deviations to the right of the bell curve of realistic results for the vast majority, or that are on growth drugs that have altered their physiology to be abnormally responsive to the stimulus of resistance exercise, or both of the above. Assuming that such individuals are simply genetic phenoms (rather than merely possessing drug-altered physiologies), then they represent the "tall trees" sticking out above the canopy that we described in the Introduction to *Body By Science*. Through relentless marketing by the bodybuilding magazines and the supplement industry, these anomalies have become the images that define the landscape for many newcomers to exercise, not realizing that such people are so far beyond the statistical norm and have next to "zero" relevance to the "forest." And that's what is empowering about our book and the truth it contains; i.e., that ours is a book that is intended as a realistic and effective exercise guideline for the forest and we reject the abnormal as being the appropriate standard by which to define normal bodybuilding, health and exercise expectations. You won't gain 30 pounds of muscle in addition to the muscle you have probably already gained from training, nor is it necessary to do so. Aim for being the best phenotype that you can fashion from your genotype, not something or somebody else.

THE NEW OLD

QUESTION: A friend of mine is a strength-training historian of sorts and he told me that he has one of the old Peary Rader strength and bodybuilding courses [Rader was the man who founded Ironman magazine in 1935]. This was long before steroids came on the scene and yet he claims that the way people trained back in those days is very close to what you are advocating now (albeit without the science to support it). According to my friend, Rader was recommending a form of abbreviated training and even a Rest-Pause style of technique and the standard workouts consisted of anywhere from one exercise to three exercises performed very infrequently. Is this true?

ANSWER: Yes it is. The interesting thing is that when you look at Peary Rader's course from the 1930s, the starting point was not a three-day-a-week routine. The starting point was a two-day a week routine and it quickly diminished to being even less frequently performed. [1] However, this was from a period of time when the water had not yet been muddied by a huge popularity of this activity to create a selection bias, and it was not muddied by the abuse of pharmaceuticals. So when you look at these courses and learn what people were doing to get good results back then, that should translate easily now. Ironically, if you really look closely at the people who have selected bodybuilding as a vocation or as a competitive sport, you will find that they have typically arrived at their decision via participation in some other activity or sport that resulted in their developing a disproportionate musculature, which, in turn, pointed out to them where their natural talent lay for bodybuilding and, consequently, inclined them to move in that direction. And that's how it tends to work in real life. That's why Bill Gates is Bill Gates and Warren Buffett is Warren Buffett. And we always find it amusing to watch business shows on television that are constantly interviewing Mr. Buffett regarding his investment advice, as, for the average person, Mr. Buffett really hasn't much relevance. He has inherent capabilities and gifts for investing that simply are not repeatable (which they should be) by the average person. If it were otherwise, then there would be a lot more Warren Buffetts running around. And this is the way it works in almost all manner of things; certain people have innate gifts or natural talent for certain things – from medicine to preaching. And this is also true with bodybuilders; they have come to strength training usually by the production of astounding results through some other activity – whether it be motocross or gymnastics -- that caused both them and the people around them to note their abnormally muscled physiques. In other words, such people have self-selected and directed themselves into this realm without the need for assistance from any "expert." Almost by definition, someone coming to a gym or a personal trainer saying that he wants to "look like a bodybuilder" is a marker for the fact that it's probably never going to happen. And the neat thing about back in the Perry Rader days is that the people who had these genetic gifts (along with the rest of society and the training philosophy of the time), did not view the pursuit of building of bigger muscles as being a license to throw away the rest of their lives and devote all of their time to this one activity. And this is an important point: if you happen to be blessed with this genetic gift, don't fall into the trap of "when your only tool is a hammer then the whole world becomes a nail," by making your training the only thing of importance in your life – because it simply is not necessary to have *that* kind of devotion to obtain the best results from bodybuilding. It's not necessary to shut off other more important areas of your life in order to pursue this goal. Top-level professional bodybuilders, to compete at the level they compete at, consume pretty much all of their income purchasing the drugs necessary to keep them at that level. The vast majority of champion bodybuilders live in efficiency apartments, sleep on futons and have a blender in their kitchen and a skillet to cook egg-whites in – and that's about it. It's not a particularly glamorous life, despite what the muscle magazines might have you believe. So if you are one of the rare few that possesses this great genetic gift of naturally big muscles, please don't use it as an excuse to squander the rest of your life.

PROFESSIONAL BODYBUILDING – AND ILL HEALTH

QUESTION: A lot of the big name bodybuilders that I grew up reading about have, for the most part, developed major health problems, usually coronary problems. And I don't know if that is just a bad statistical analysis in that these are conditions that they would have developed anyway as a natural course of things (just as many people in the general population do), but it seems odd to me. I saw the DVD of the reunion of the stars of the film Pumping Iron, *all of who were top bodybuilders from the 70s– and they looked awful; frail, skinny, sickly. Many of them looked like they never lifted a weight in their lives. By contrast, I recall seeing former Mr. Universe John Grimek when he was in his 70s and he still looked great – and was still very strong. Is this just a random statistical variation or are we starting to see now the coming home to roost of the anabolic drug abuses that occurred with bodybuilders from the 70s?*

ANSWER: We suspect that the ill health that you (and others) have witnessed in these former champions is a result that occurred partly from their drug use and partly from the degree of overtraining that was going on in that era. The 1970s marked the first time that there was an adequate amount of drugs to actually ignore or try to violate the rules of nature in terms of human recovery ability. And the ill health that developed in these former champions may simply have been a consequence of their chronic, unrelenting overtraining. After all, the things that will accelerate the aging and disease process are oxidative damage and over-nutrition. Or, stated conversely, the things that seem to prolong life span and extend youth appear to be limitations of oxidative damage and caloric intake (or intermittent fasting). The overtraining that occurred during this era, when combined with the six-meals-a-day food consumption that was the norm, when coupled with their bodies' attempt to stay in an on-going positive nitrogen balance actually served to produce a chronic inflammatory state that, in our opinion, served to greatly accelerate the rate of atherosclerotic disease (heart disease, stroke, cancers, etc.). These bodybuilders were training so much, and for such prolonged periods of time, and producing so much oxidative damage and suffering from so much over nutrition and drug usage that it eventually led to ill health (please recall our definition of health and the role of appropriate balance between the catabolic and anabolic states). Many bodybuilders have died, and many more look like they're on their last legs – and these were individuals who once possessed awesomely impressive physiques. And we, like most people who saw them, once looked to them as people who "had to know" what they were talking about regarding muscle building, health and fitness because of the apparent condition of their great physiques. Fast-forwarding to present day, we're saddened to see that many of these bodybuilders are either in terrible shape or dead.

A CAREER IN PROFESSIONAL BODYBUILDING: YEA OR NAY?

QUESTION: *Knowing this, if a young man came to you saying he was interested in bodybuilding and wanted to be a competitive bodybuilder (and thought he had the potential for it), would you recommend that he "go for it?"*

ANSWER: We would honestly tell this young man not to do it. And the reason is that bodybuilding (at the competitive level) is nothing more than a beauty contest. We're talking about a man going on stage in bikini underwear, slathered in oil, with muscles that have been temporarily pumped up backstage and striking poses – and that's all it is. Moreover, bodybuilding competition is actually more bizarre than your average beauty contest because it is a beauty contest that quickly morphs into something that is really strange, because what gives you a competitive advantage in a bodybuilding competition is anything that stands out as unusual or extreme. The result being that this pursuit actually evolves into something that is not physiologically functional or healthy in any possible way. Particularly with the way that bodybuilding is now, it has turned into something that is an unrealistic freak show that is not open to the vast majority of the genotypes that exist. And even for the ones that it is open to, it has been abused to such an extreme level that we think that it automatically qualifies as an unhealthy activity. So our inclination would be to say, "don't do it." Now, having said that, the activity of "building" one's "body" is a very healthful activity and its benefits are readily available to any and all who partake of it. Indeed, the results that were produced by average people back in the Peary Rader days were actually quite impressive and quite astounding. And we think that is what should be strived for. To most of the people that have read *Body By Science* we would suggest that they not ever pick up a muscle magazine. They will be better served by setting up a primitive setup in their garage than going to most commercial gyms because the distractions and the misinformation that they will encounter in these environments is very counter productive.

GENETIC VARIATIONS

QUESTIONS: *Is it ever desirable to change the routine you have listed?*

ANSWER: Yes, and have indicated in *Body By Science* why this may be necessary and how to do so. There is another reason, however, which has to do with the different genetic markers (which we covered in some detail in Chapter Four of *Body By Science*). Enzymatic markers such as interleukin 15, ciliary neurotrophic factor, alpha-actin-3 (among other genetic markers) can all effect how and to what degree a given individual will respond to resistance exercise in terms of varying levels of both the volume and frequency of his training. The problem inherent in any exercise prescription is that it is very hard to determine such genetic factors in advance, or even by empirical experimentation, owing to the fact that such factors are not typically expressed homogeneously throughout the body, as different combinations of these genetic components may be more or less prevalent throughout different muscle groups on a given individual. Apart from this problem, there exist two more; one is the problem of selection bias and the other is the problem of face validity. "Selection bias" refers to the "tall trees" analogy that we referred to in Chapter One of *Body By Science*, and speaks to the fact that the individuals with the best genetic markers for excelling at a given activity will be the ones who typically will excel at a given activity, far surpassing the majority of us in terms of potential and physical capability. It is in our nature to gravitate to such people for advice, even when they do not necessarily have any relevant advice to give. Consequently, the waters become muddied by the fact that such people can do anything and everything – yet still display tremendous results, rendering their "how to" advice meaningless (as it is tantamount to saying that everything works equally well, which, when viewed from this context, is palpably false). In other words, the investment advice that Warren Buffet has to give us is probably not nearly as relevant as the advice that Ben Stein has to give us. And what Ben Stein recommends is to start while you're young and invest in an index fund, putting a little in each month – and then don't worry about it. And what Ben Stein says about investing is what we say about training; i.e., pick out a good, comprehensive training routine that covers the basics and covers all the major muscle groups in your body, limit your volume, limit your frequency and emphasize your recovery and you're going to get the best results possible. When you start micro-managing your workouts, that's when you're likely to run into problems. This being said, we recognize that we do not have genetics on our side of the ledger; i.e., those with exceptional genetics are already extremely well developed and muscular, and, consequently, they do not seek out a better way to train their bodies, as a "better way" has never been necessary for them. The people who desire a better way are typically those who are not satisfied with their present level of development (i.e., those of modest genetics), and consequently they are the ones that require whatever edge science can give them. Such trainees will grow bigger and stronger, but most of them will never achieve the results of those "taller" trees in the forest and, consequently, many will grow frustrated with any training approach they employ, as no training method can deliver results that one's genetics do not allow. And beckoning from the sidelines will be those individuals that display superior results that say, "Here's how *I* did it." And we have to acknowledge that they *do* have the genetically superior results and that whatever method they employed is, in fact, *how* they did it. And, indeed, there may exist a small sub-segment within the general population that will find that what we're advocating may not produce optimal gains for them or, even if it does apply, there will be some who will simply not choose to employ it to their full benefit, with the result that we do need to acknowledge that there may be a problem with compliance. In terms of "face validity," that selection bias in favor of the genetically gifted trainee always exists to challenge what we recommend because we are unable to offer up sufficient superior examples to successfully challenge the genetic marvels. Moreover, the face validity of high-intensity training has often been damaged by the very ones who were (and are) its strongest advocates. For instance, during the 1980s books detailing high-intensity training experiments in which subjects who had great genetics for building muscle and had been heavy users of steroids were taken off their frequently performed high volume, lower intensity workouts and put on high-intensity training programs (it was also believed that they were taken off steroids at this time) and, quite clearly, they looked worse for the experience. Such individuals harken back to our chapter in *Body By Science* that detailed the different genetic components that factor into an individual's response to the exercise stimulus (such as interleukin 15). Such individuals are rare, but they do exist. The reader will recall that there was one genotype, and it was homozygous, that was able to produce a large increase in muscle mass but very little change in strength, which means that this person may not have any measurable recording to show progress in the gym, yet still produce considerable muscle growth. The opposite genotype (or the homozygous in the opposite direction) is indicated in individuals that can produce very significant increases in strength with very minimal increases in size. In the failed high-intensity examples cited above, we had individuals that, on their workout records, were able to show excellent progress in strength, but little to no appreciable progress in the mirror. This may be a result of the fact that, from a genetics standpoint, muscle growth, the cosmetic portion that everyone is seeking, may actually be an adaptation of "last resort" based upon one's genotype, meaning that if one can produce changes in strength through enzymatic or neurological means, then one's body will preferentially do this because that, to one's body, is a lower-order investment. But if one is of a genotype that makes one unable to produce such lower-order investments, one will default to hypertrophy as a means of increasing strength. And that's borne out in the data on interleukin-15; those that produced the best hypertrophy response produced the worst strength response and vice versa. In light of this, the muscular growth process may well be a process of last resort in any case owing to its great metabolic cost. It may be that after one has tapped out one's enzymatic adaptations and one's neurological adaptations, that one's body will resort to a size adaptation. And this may be why most people observe that they have a progression in strength that is then later followed by a mass increase. By the same token, there exists a subset of the population that has the opposite reaction; i.e., they get bigger and *then* they get stronger. Indeed, Internet forums are replete with people calling each other names, each accusing the other of misrepresenting the "truth" about training, when, in fact, they are both telling the truth. The vast majority of trainees we see typically gain strength before they gain muscle size because from a biological standpoint that is the most economic way for the body to adapt. But there are other genotypes where the opposite is true; they have the opposite type of interlukin-15 variation whereby they gain size and then revert to a strength gain as a result of the size gain. So some people may register such that the size gain comes first, and then later registers a strength gain, but we believe that a larger portion of the population first exhausts other mechanisms of improving strength and then, as a last resort, produces more muscle tissue. And then, in a similar vein, there may even be a small sub-segment of the population that are simply non-responders to any type of training – period (and this would include the type of training that we advocate). Nevertheless, if one keeps accurate workout records one can go a long way towards determining one's response (or lack thereof) to a given modality of training. The questions one should ask oneself would be:

Am I getting stronger?
Are my measurements improving?
Is my body composition improving?
Do I feel good more days than I feel spent?

This last point is important as there's going to be a down period after a workout where one's functional capability is lower than baseline, and the more advanced one becomes in one's training, the more one can feel this. And for most people (just like it averaged out in the Nautilus North Study), it is our experience from having trained thousands of clients over a period of 15-years that, across the board, most people are going to find their optimal training frequency to be once every seven days. There will be some outliers that can tolerate training every two to three days, and there will be some outliers that can only train but once every twelve to fourteen days. However, training once a week is a good starting point to try and parse out the outliers. What we've learned is that if one keeps good workout records, and makes minor changes to volume and frequency throughout a period of many months (both up and down the volume and frequency scale), when one looks back on one's training records over a period of two or three years one will begin to see patterns of progress emerging or receding during these periods of change. This provides the trainee with an aerial view that will give him a sense of what it is he should be doing and, consequently, what his genotype may be for optimizing the training stimulus. The "Big 5" workout that we have recommended in "Body By Science," however, remains an excellent starting point for all trainees and then, if necessary, adjustments can be made from this baseline program. And if one has access to a good, objective measurement device (such as a Bod Pod) this can give one lots of additional and authentic data that one can then act upon.

MUSCLE GROWTH –
A SLOW PROCESS

QUESTION: Why is the muscle building process so slow?

ANSWER: Simply because we evolved as a creature that lived in an environment of food scarcity. In our natural environment food was scarce and one had to expend a lot of energy to acquire it. And once acquired, its caloric density was quite low. Muscle is very important for survival. If you can't move efficiently and effectively, one can't obtain food and one can't keep from becoming food. But above a certain level of musculature, it quickly develops a point of diminishing returns because muscle is metabolically expensive tissue. And beyond a certain point there are strong negative regulators of muscle growth, as the body doesn't don't want to add on this tissue unnecessarily because of the metabolic demands it places on the body. As a consequence, there has to be a really strong stimulus that's going to say to the organism, "Hey, this tissue is necessary and it is worth the metabolic sacrifice to have it." In other words, the reason that muscle is so hard to acquire is that it is a metabolically expensive tissue and we evolved as a creature that can't afford high levels of metabolic expense.

REALISTIC EXPECTATIONS

QUESTION: Realistically, how much muscle can be gained in the course of one year, in terms of pure muscle?

ANSWER: The response side of the equation is going to be highly variable and dictated by genetics. But if one were to spread all of the possible responses out on a bell-shaped curve and you were to go right down the middle of the bell and look at the average response that someone could expect with proper training over the course of training career, we believe it would be possible to gain between 18 and 20 pounds of muscle. Now this would be based upon the average subject who was starting resistance training and realizing his genetic potential. There will be people who will say, "That doesn't sound like very much!" But you've got to remember that our expectations of what a good response is have been entirely warped. If, for instance, we look at contemporary bodybuilders, they're taking very good genetics and pouring on top of that very large amounts of anabolic steroids and very large amounts of growth hormone. And you're seeing these 250-270 pound competitors with single digit body fat that are winning contests. And that has hugely skewed our expectation of what a "good gain" is. If you want to, say, take an average person and add 18 to 20 pounds of muscle on their frames over the course of a year – which is possible – and you say, "Well, that's not *that* great." Go to the grocery store and pick up a pound of ground beef and then get to the corner of the meat counter and stack up 18 of those and look at what that actually is. And imagine that put onto the frame of an average person -- that's an astounding amount of muscle. Non-steroid studies reveal that the amount of muscle that someone can gain once they have exited puberty is *not* massive. However, it may grow to be significant over time, but certainly in the short term – say the first five months or so, you might be looking at four, five or six pounds, which in all honesty is a fairly considerable amount of muscle. Guys should be happy if they can gain five pounds and women needn't worry that they are going to gain 40 pounds. By the same token, most of the studies conducted on muscle growth have been relatively short term and when we've looked at the protocols being used, the amount of muscle that one could expect to gain in such a short period of time had to be fairly modest. While that's true across the board, if you bring a good protocol to your workout you can expect a little bit better than that in most subjects, although it will probably still be modest. However, if you put on even a modest amount of muscle on an average individual, and if you pay enough attention to diet where you strip away the overlying bodyfat, the effect of that can be incredibly dramatic. You can gain five or eight pounds of muscle and get your body fat down to nine or 10 percent and that, on a male, is a combination that can produce an appearance change that looks like a 25 or 30 pound muscle increase.

CALF TRAINING

QUESTION: *I've tried to add size to my calves for three years now and have tried all sorts of training methods, including running every day. My calves haven't grown an inch. What gives?*

ANSWER: The calf muscle is a muscle that is not open to a lot of growth and hypertrophy – for several reasons. One reason is its geometry, as the shape and length of its musculotendinous unit is relatively fixed. Another reason is that the muscles underneath the gastrocnemius (which serve to determine its shape and potential size), such as the soleus muscle, are pinnate muscles that, because of their geometry are not muscles that can hypertrophy to any meaningful level. And finally, the calf is a muscle that is involved in continuous weight bearing and typically has a very low content of fast-twitch (hypertrophy prone) fibers, which are the ones with the greatest mass potential in the body. If the calves are overtrained, such as they would have been with your running every day, whatever growth potential your calves might have would have been prevented from being realized. Consequently, no matter what one's training regimen is going to be, it's going to be bound and limited by these components, the biggest being the simple geometry of the muscle group itself. In terms of the musculotendinous unit, the majority of the population has quite a long Achilles tendon attachment relative to a fairly short gastrocnemius muscle.

MCGUFF'S ANAMNESTIC WORKOUT EXPERIENCE

QUESTION: *On Dr. McGuff's website he has an article in which he discussed an anamnestic approach to exercise. It seems that he was recommending training a little more frequently than once a week and I was curious if he is still doing that?*

ANSWER: The idea for the anamnestic response is an idea that came from the field of immunology. It is the same idea that underlies the reasons for getting a booster shot; i.e., a second application of a stimulus in a short span of time that ramps up the adaptive response in the immune system. It was an interesting theory and one that looked to have legs, as in his workout performed on the second day Doug's strength gains were much greater, but after the second or third round of such workouts retrogression started to become evident as a result of overtraining and any and all progress soon ground to a halt. According to Dr. McGuff:

> I now believe that the early improvement that I saw with those second day workouts is what is referred to as "synaptic facilitation." And this is when basically the neuro-motor pathways of recruiting motor units for those particular movements had been primed by the previous days' work. So on the second round, your motor unit recruitment and motor unit firing rate were now more efficient. Consequently, the apparent increases in strength at that time were more of a neurological efficiency or a neurological priming from the first workout. In other words, the increases in strength were not sustainable, as even by the third round of training in such a fashion the accumulative effects of overtraining from it obviated any improvement in neurological efficiency and it all became a wash. So it was more of a theoretical experiment, but given enough time it didn't pan out at all. It may have some limited application as a means of tweaking the training stimulus for trainees that have reached mechanical sticking points in their movements; like if you've got them on the chest press and they can't progress because they have reached a mechanical sticking point. At this point you could use

an anamnestic workout (i.e., a second, back-to-back workout) to engage that enhanced motor unit recruitment efficiency, which will help to get them over their sticking point so that they can continue to progress weight. But you should reserve it for certain little tricks like that, not as an on-going technique.

-- Doug McGuff, MD

HIGH-INTENSITY: A DIFFERENT SPECIES OF EXERCISE

QUESTION: High-intensity training would appear to be a different "species" of exercise when compared to other modalities such as walking, golf, jogging, etc. Why does high-intensity training produce such dramatic effects on the body?

ANSWER: You have to think of high-intensity exercise within its proper context; i.e., from an evolutionary standpoint. And when viewed in this light you have to ask yourself how infrequently – in terms of volume and frequency – would such a level of intensity typically be encountered by an organism during its day-to-day existence? If one is a hunter-gatherer, for example, one is going to have a big kill that's going to be of a high-intensity nature and will require one to induce a high level of muscular fatigue, but then one will have an adequate respite from it in that one is not going to be volitionally putting oneself in that position again until the opportunity presents itself. By contrast, in the fitness industry, for people who are trying to either lose bodyfat or gain muscle (or both), there is so much neurosis involved and that neurosis is exploited for commercial purposes. No matter what publication you pick up everything within its pages is designed to create training angst in the subject. So there's always this push to try the "next new thing" or "push the volume" or this thing's "good," this thing's "bad." The problem is that a lot of times what we are wanting to get is a response out of our bodies that we're seeing out of someone with a completely different genetic makeup from us.

MYOSTATIN SUPPLEMENTS

QUESTION: I have heard that some supplements can be myostatin blockers. What are your thoughts on this?

ANSWER: After the significance of myostatin became known to the bodybuilding world it didn't take long for supplement companies to put out their own "myostatin blockers" which were predicated on the cystoseira canariensis molecule, which is a component in seaweed that was found to bind myostatin. The problem was that it did bind myostatin in vitro (in a test tube), but in vivo it had no activity whatsoever owing to the fact that it bound the handle portion of the "key" but not the ridges on the key. A study was conducted by Dave Willoughby, [2] in which he examined the alleged efficacy of this supplement and he concluded that it did nothing. Still, since supplement companies have very little to do with science (particularly when there is money to be made), more supplements came out. And since the supplement business is largely unregulated, the supplement manufacturers made all sorts of false and unsubstantiated claims about the potency of their myostatin blocking supplements. And these supplement companies rode a huge wave of income production for six to nine months until it became readily apparent to everyone that their products simply didn't work. And this speaks to a point made in our Introduction to *Body By Science*; i.e., that there are both honest mistakes and willful deception in the fitness industry. The real danger in this is that the greater the likelihood for honest error in our understanding, the greater the opportunity that exists for deliberate deception. And the areas where we're most likely to deceive ourselves are exactly the areas where someone can take the opportunity to defraud us.

MUSCLE:
THE UNAPPRECIATED GIFT

QUESTION: I'm really interested in getting stronger for all the reasons that your book indicates. However, I have a problem in that I gain muscle size very easily. Unlike many trainees, I have absolutely "zero" desire to get any bigger. I'm very intrigued by the scientific nature of your "Big 5" program, but is there a way that I could do it that would prevent me from gaining any more muscle size?

ANSWER: In all the years that the authors have been training clients we've had perhaps five people who would be classified as really strong responders in terms of expressing the potential to build large amounts of muscle mass. And, without exception, we can tell you that the ones that have this capability don't care about it and don't want it. And while we can alter the protocol so that it will be less friendly to muscle growth, our suspicion is that any level of meaningful exertion by these people is going to produce a fairly large increase in muscle mass. It's ironic that the people that have this genetic gift don't want it and the people that don't have it seem to crave it – but we've never encountered someone who has the gift that actually wants to actualize it. It's a very strange phenomenon. And women of course have other factors that militate against their bodies producing bigger muscles, such as a lack of testosterone, which is a major component in building muscle mass. Consequently, insufficient testosterone levels serve to prevent females from developing massive muscles no matter how hard or how heavy they train. And what we're finding (and what the scientific literature is slowly starting to bear out) is that certain hormones that have anabolic effects, like testosterone and growth hormone, are found to have upstream effects on Myostatin. So while testosterone, per se, factors into the production of muscle tissue, muscle growth itself is related to Myostatin. For instance, increasing the amount of growth hormone in the body will have an inhibitory effect on the production of Myostatin, with the result that as growth hormone levels rise, Myostatin production falls. In other words, the hormonal effects on muscle mass that we're seeing are actually upstream effects that effect levels of Myostatin in the bloodstream. And what this fact points to is that it is your level of Myostatin expression that is ultimately going to determine when your improvement curve, in terms of muscle size, is going to become asymptotic and start to level out. But just because that is occurring does not mean that you are cut off from all of the other beneficial effects that appropriate high-intensity exercise can bring you in terms of enhanced functional ability and overall health.

STEROIDS

QUESTION: Steroids are so much in the news these days. And the general assumption now is that if an individual has large muscles, he probably is "on something." However, I've never really seen a paper that relates what it is that steroids actually do. I know from observation that when people go off steroids they get smaller, and that leads me to believe that there is very little actual tissue being produced. I've also noted that since muscle is over 76% water, perhaps there is a greater retention of water when one is on steroids. And then when one no longer is on them, he no longer has that lightning rod in his muscles to draw water into them and the water simply gets flushed out. But by the same token, the athletes who take the drugs appear to be stronger, so there must be some sort of tissue building going on. What are your thoughts on this?

ANSWER: Well, our thoughts used to be along the lines of what you said, but those thoughts came out of the Arthur Jones/Nautilus era assertion that steroids really did not work. And the problem with this position was it just didn't pass the sniff test; because you would see people use steroids and their muscles would get a lot bigger. So the Nautilus position simply lacked "face validity," which is simply a medical phrase meaning that, on the face of it, it seemed like bullshit. What steroids actually do is get transported within a cell and work on its DNA machinery to increase the transcriptional rate of contractile proteins – actin, myosin, myosin heavy chains, myosin light chains – all of the things that serve to increase the volume of muscle cells – are going to also have an upstream effect that will result in diminishing one's Myostatin expression and, therefore, will result in the production of more muscle mass. So, yes, steroids really do work. Our discussion then becomes when you go off steroids, why does the muscle that you built up go away? Well, because when you go off of steroids the exact opposite happens; you've got to remember that these hormones are all regulated by a complex feedback mechanism. The simplest way of explaining it is to liken it to the thermostat in your house when the air conditioner is on; if you set your thermostat at 74 degrees and the cool air starts coming into the room, as soon as the room temperature drops to 73 degrees the thermostat shuts the air conditioner off. In this respect, your hypothalamus, your pituitary, as well as your androgenic hormones are regulated from the level of your hypothalamus, which releases gonadotrophin releasing factors to your pituitary, which releases hormones which then stimulate your adrenal gland and testes to release these hormones. But think about what happens if you have a house with the thermostat set and all of a sudden you exogenously pump in a bunch of cold air such that the temperature of the room drops down to 60 degrees? Well, when you stop pumping in that cold air, there is going to be a long period before the thermostat kicks back on again. Similarly, when you have been taking exogenous steroids for a long period of time, your hypothalamus and your pituitary – like the thermostat -- simply shut down. And if you use steroids for a period of longer than five to seven days, these glands then assume that the exogenous material will be oncoming, and shut down completely. And they will not kick back in for a prolonged period of time after the exogenous material is taken away. So if someone has been taking exogenous steroids for a period of months and then stops, he's going to have "zero" endogenous androgenic hormone production for a period of months. And he will experience massive muscle wasting as a result because in the same way that there was an upstream effect on Myostatin levels while taking the steroid (thus limiting the amount of Myostatin in his body), when that upstream effect is removed, then there is an increased Myostatin expression and very significant muscle wasting. And this is where Arthur Jones probably ran into trouble when he tried to take professional bodybuilders and demonstrate how brief, high-intensity training could be more effective for these bodybuilders. When he got them to come to Nautilus to train, he had a very strict policy that steroids would *not* be taken, but he also had a very strong belief that they did not work. And he probably did not have an understanding of how the hypothalamic pituitary axis of these bodybuilders would be inhibited for months upon months. So, for instance, in 1983 when he brought in Boyer Coe and had him stop using steroids, when you look at the *Nautilus Advanced Bodybuilding Book* and you look at Boyer Coe, rather than looking better than he did on steroids, he looked gaunt and skinny. Ellington Darden once spoke about the plans they had for champion bodybuilder Eddie Robinson to do a similar sort of program, the purpose of which was to demonstrate how a very brief – twice a week – program of high-intensity training could really produce the best results for him. But they couldn't get any results out of his body at all because when they took him in to have his serum testosterone levels tested *they were not even detectable*. And the reason was that he had stopped taking steroids, which was the policy at Nautilus at the time, and, consequently, his body was not producing any testosterone whatsoever. So he was in a hormonal state where it was simply *impossible* for him to gain muscle regardless of the type of training he was engaged in. So, again, steroids do work while you're taking them, but the flip side of that is that you're going to have a problem when you stop taking them because you're not going to have any of your own endogenous production left after taking supra-normal levels of those hormones.

GYNECOMASTIA AND GONAD SHRINKAGE

QUESTION: I've heard that many bodybuilders that use steroids develop breasts and their gonads shrink! Is this true – or just a myth?

ANSWER: It's true. The breast development is a medical condition that develops from taking anabolic steroids, as there are enzymes within the body that act upon androgenic hormones and that serve to push them down a metabolic pathway towards estrogen. And this is when you see bodybuilding competitors that experience shrinkage of their gonads and the development of Gynecomastia ("bitch tits"). This is a result of their bodies' testosterone levels being so exongenously high that they end up being pushed down these metabolic pathways where they end up being esterified into estrogens and they then develop secondary female sex characteristics along with these conditions. The gonad shrinkage is a direct result of supply and demand; i.e., you're having shrinkage of that tissue for the very reason that it's not having to produce testosterone if you're receiving it synthetically or exongenously. That is one reason for the shrinkage. Another reason is the supra-normal levels of the androgenic hormones are now being metabolized to estrogens and, thus, produce an additional inhibitory effect as well. And, we might add, if someone is taking high levels of hormones, then all bets are off regarding the efficacy of any training program one might be on because one will have completely changed the environment of the organism and its response to training. And you may also be changing what program may be most efficacious by steroid ingestion.

STEROIDS AND HEALTH DANGERS

QUESTION: The health dangers of steroids – are they real or overstated?

ANSWER: The answer is that the dangers are *both* real and overstated. Things such as "roid rage" and psychosis to some extent has been overplayed. The major media event that surrounded the death of professional wrestler Chris Benoit, an individual who happened to take steroids during his career, is an example of this. Such a simplistic response (i.e., "steroids did it") fails to factor into the equation the types of narcissistic personality disorders that go into those kinds of sports and occupations, along with a little bit of elevated testosterone levels. Mix into this the frustration that attends not being able to go off of steroids owing to their role in the appearance you require for your profession. And then there's the frustration of living with the reality that, despite how it appears on TV, such professions as wrestling are an incredibly unreliable way to earn a living. All of these things are stressors that can create situations that can result in such tragedy. But to blame it solely on steroid use strikes us as being too simplistic. Now, having said this, there are health risks to exogenous steroids, one of which is that steroid hormones are also intrinsically involved with cholesterol metabolism, and it can alter things in such a way that you have increased arteriosclerotic deposits, which could mean that you're going to have an increased risk for heart attack, stroke and things of this nature. And mineralicorticoids or corticoid steroids can have other effects on things such as blood sugar levels (which will have diabetic type expression), as well as effects on water and sodium retention, which can result in hypertension – all events that have definite health consequences. And then there are certain types of tumors (particularly those that give rise to prostate cancer) that have testosterone receptors. Consequently, if you happen to have a small prostatic nodule that's lying dormant and that's not going to turn into cancer until you're 58-years old, but all of a sudden you're ingesting a lot of exogenous steroids, this tiny tumor (that is testosterone receptor sensitive) will all of a sudden ramp up. So there are some health consequences but we don't think they are of any sort of magnitude to justify congressional hearings like we've been having. Nevertheless, and while we're on the topic of steroids, it should be remembered that steroids are also produced out of the adrenal gland. And the adrenal gland is like a nut with three different layers; a cortex, a medial or middle layer, and a medulla or central layer, and the pneumonic used in medical school is "Salt, Sugar, Sex – the deeper you go the better it gets." The outer layer is salt (the mineralacorticoids), the middle layer is glucocorticoids (which control sugar related things), and then the sex steroid hormones are located in the central portion, so you can see anatomically where these hormones are produced; they go from one zone to the next. And these are very closely related and can be metabolized in such a way that they can be interchangeable. So you're not just going to have an isolated effect when using a steroid. And this is true of any drug. and it's also true of exercise. No drug has a single effect; all drugs have potential toxic effects and they're going to interact with other drugs, and this is true of steroids as well.

STEROIDS AND AGING

QUESTION: *I have noted that for years those who took steroids seemed to age quicker than those who did not. People who took them while in their teens soon looked like they were in their mid twenties; those who took them in their twenties, soon looked as though they were in their thirties, and so on. Is it possible that aging can be accelerated by steroid ingestion?*

ANSWER: A lot of male aging in particular is driven by testosterone. For instance, going from adolescence into adulthood, the rise in testosterone that occurs in adolescence is involved with the extension of growth plates and the closing of growth plates, where cartilage turns into bone. And other characteristics that you see with aging are mediated by testosterone receptors; for instance, male pattern baldness, facial hair that becomes evident as you grow older – growing hair in your nose and ears—those are all testosterone receptor issues. And exogenous steroids, because you're going to have a surplus of this stuff floating around, are going to start to bind those receptors and you're going to get those secondary characteristics that you normally don't see until you become much older.

ROID RAGE

QUESTION: *I'm intrigued by the issue of "roid rage." Is this real? Can steroids really affect the brain?*

ANSWER: Steroids can affect the brain. The brain is filled with testosterone receptors and the functioning of the brain, and the differentiation of the brain en utero, is driven to a large extent by the hormonal environment, and whether it's testosterone or estrogen dominant. This is why, despite the best pacifist intentions of almost every parent in our current society, the average three to five year old boy -- across the board -- will display incredibly bellicose traits and characteristics. You can take a child who has never been exposed to a handgun and he will fashion a weapon out of anything he can find; he'll pick a stick up and turn it into a knife, a bayonet, a handgun, a rifle -- and this is just "testosterone in action" in the developing brain. There is some support that rage could come from that sort of thing, although we don't know if there is strong scientific evidence to support it, and even if there is we still think that through the popular media it is hugely overstated.

BODYFAT LEVELS INCREASING WITH MUSCLE MASS INCREASES

QUESTION: Years ago I a read an interview that was conducted with Dr. Barbara Hansen, a specialist in primate research as it pertains to diabetes in which she said that it's almost impossible to not gain fat when you gain muscle because there's a thin fatty membrane within a muscle cell, and therefore when you gain muscle you are to some extent going to be increasing your bodyfat. Does this make sense?

ANSWER: Yes this makes sense, although the cell membrane she is referring to is only made up of a layer two lipids thick. Fat has a hydrophilic head (meaning a "water loving" head) and a hydrophobic tail. And the outside of a cell is bathed in water, and the inside of it is bathed in water. So you get a lipid bilayer that makes up the cell membrane. And what that means is that you have two layers of fat that line up their hydrophobic tails with each other and therefore project their hydrophilic or water loving heads to the exterior or interior of the cell. This, then, is what makes up a cell membrane, but she is correct; if you're going to add additional tissue, you're going to have a cell membrane which is made up of fat – but, again, that fat is only two molecules thick for each cell, which doesn't add up to much -- especially when compared to the amount of lipid molecules stored in a single fat globual.

GAINING MUSCLE EASIER WHEN YOU GAIN FAT

QUESTION: Is it easier to gain muscle when you're well nourished and perhaps even gaining some fat than it is when you're dieting to lose fat?

ANSWER: We've found that, to some degree, an increase in one's level of bodyfat often times makes the metabolic environment more permissive for muscle growth. And, from an economic/biological standpoint, if you are going to add tissue that has a significant caloric expense, the ease of adding that tissue is going to be permitted by the addition of some additional stored energy, and perhaps that's why the growth of skeletal muscle does tend to correlate with an increase in one's body fat. It's easier to gain muscle when you are "bulking," because the two kind of go hand in hand, in that muscle mass increases are permitted by slightly higher levels of body fat as you are carrying with you an extra caloric requirement that the addition of this metabolically expensive tissue might require. By the same token, the converse is also true; when you are losing body fat it is hard to gain muscle simultaneously – not impossible, but hard -- because if the caloric restriction is too severe, not only are you going to be tapping your fat reserves, but your body will also want to cut its overhead. In this respect, your body is just like a corporation; i.e., if the caloric input drops too precipitously, that is to say, too fast for you to tap into body fat reserves, there's also going to be a powerful biological message to jettison some skeletal muscle because of its metabolic expense in the face of a caloric deficit. So we think that if you're dieting to get cut (defined), it's almost impossible not to lose some lean tissue because your body is trying to cut overhead expense.

PART THREE:
SPECIAL NEEDS

PROBLEMS WITH TYPICAL PHYSIOTHERAPY TREATMENTS

QUESTION: What are the actual requirements for a genuine rehabilitation from an injury? Many physiotherapists simply give their patients a photocopied sheet with several exercises on it, of which they might check off three or four that the patient should perform (as not all of the exercises on the sheet have applicability). And they typically do this once the allowed insurance treatment is over.

ANSWER: You'll find that what happens under most physical therapy circumstances is that the frequency and volume of the work that's being done is dictated largely by what the insurance companies will pay for, rather than any objective measure of what needs to be done. For instance, an insurance company may, during the first five weeks of rehab, provide for five days a week of rehab treatment (conveniently scheduled from Monday through Friday), as if the body follows a physiologic basis based on the five-day work week. And these treatments may occur for two to three weeks, at which point the patient is sent home with a sheet of exercises to do. But after that, the patient is more or less cut loose. A more effective rehab might have required the patient to perform special exercises starting out at twice a week, and then cutting back to once a week, and carried out over a much longer span of time (and incorporated with a good general conditioning program). However, since that's not the way that the insurance companies have set themselves up to be paid, such considerations are seldom what should be done to produce optimal rehabilitation results for the patient. It's the "golden rule" in action, which is, simply stated, "that he who holds the gold makes the rules" – as opposed to anything objective. Even the training advice proffered by rehab specialists seems spurious, as they will often advise a patient to perform certain stretches and rehab exercises in some instances up to four times a day. How one can strengthen – if that's what these exercises are really for – the supporting musculature without progressive resistance and without paying attention to the issues of recovery and overcompensation is never indicated. Such factors become even more relevant when dealing with issues such as lower back pain, problem joints and tendons in which inflammation is present and that actually require protracted periods of rest as part of their rehabilitation.

STRETCHING – A SECOND LOOK

QUESTION: In Chapter 10 of Body By Science *you examined many of the myths that have surrounded the activity of stretching. Since this activity has been shown to diminish strength and not enhance one's range or flexibility, why do most physiotherapists continue to advocate it?*

ANSWER: That is a question that might best be addressed by the physiotherapists that you mention. We would add that even if stretching yielded some benefit, the fact remains that placing a muscle in its weakest position (the position where it can least accommodate the application of external force) and then applying force to it is an invitation to a muscle or tendon strain, and stretching a muscle, tendon or joint that is inflamed only serves to exacerbate (not diminish) the symptoms. Moreover, what a lot of physiotherapists presume to be "stretching exercises" are actually nothing more than activities that produce a state of active or passive insufficiency in the muscles involved. For instance, you've no doubt seen an individual take hold of his ankle and pull it up to his buttocks in the belief that this is "stretching" his quadriceps – but what he is actually doing is producing insufficiency; i.e., he has fully contracted his hamstring muscles to the point where the muscles in his quadriceps no longer have enough mechanical purchase to be able to contract. This produces a tugging or pulling sensation in the quadriceps muscle, but in terms of the range of motion of that muscle, such an activity does nothing to enhance its range of motion or flexibility. Instead, it simply produces a tugging, pulling, tearing sensation. The same situation exists with what is popularly referred to as the "hurdler's stretch," in which one places one's quadriceps in a fully contracted position with a flexed hip, so that the hamstring muscle is unable to initiate a contraction. This, also, produces a tugging sensation, but, again, it is not doing anything to enhance flexibility around the knee or the hip joint. The general public and rehabilitation community mistakenly confuse such activities as stretching, but it's simply placing a lengthened muscle in a position where it cannot contract -- either because of overwhelming force or a mechanical disadvantage -- and this serves no real benefit at all. True stretching requires the application of force at the extremes of a safe range of motion. And under rehab conditions this might be relatively constrained, but, nevertheless, over time that restrained range of motion will expand as strengthening occurs. So, by definition, if one is set appropriately in a strength training machine during normal circumstances (where range of motion is full) or, during rehab circumstances (where range of motion is restricted to what is tolerable to the injured area), one has, by definition, provided appropriate stretching to the area in question. Nevertheless, most rehabilitation specialists (even those that deal with professional athletes and, thus, multi-million dollar careers) have ignored the rehabilitation benefits of proper progressive resistance exercise in favor of comparatively inefficient modalities such as passive and active insufficiency activities. This, unfortunately, is done to the detriment of the patient seeking rehabilitation for his or her injuries.

LOWER BACK PAIN: SYMPTOM RELIEF VS REHABILITATION

QUESTION: What can I do to rehabilitate chronic lower back pain? I've been to chiropractors and massage therapists but the fact that I've been doing this for two years suggests that they really haven't been that effective.

ANSWER: The most common ailment we see in our facilities is lower back pain. Fortunately, it has been our experience that the majority of lower back problems tend to be self-correcting. However, this phenomenon makes it problematic in stating with certainty that "this" procedure or rehabilitative treatment caused "that" symptomatic relief response. In addition, many alleged back "treatments" are effective in treating the symptoms of lower back pain but not the underlying cause. Such treatments, particularly when viewed in the light of the self-correcting nature of the majority of lower back ailments, does next to nothing to actually protect the patient or client from future flare ups of the same condition. It is important to understand that lower back pain is extraordinarily common. Yes, it can be very debilitating (at least on a short-term basis), but everything in the Emergency Medicine literature supports the position that in the vast majority of cases it doesn't really matter what is done to treat lower back pain, as most problems will self-correct in a 6-to-12-week period. Consequently, the fact that someone has had apparent success in relieving the symptoms of his lower back pain by seeing a chiropractor, a massage therapist, an acupuncturist or even a physiotherapist, doesn't necessarily mean that these modalities really did anything at all. However, given that even after such "treatments" the condition still exists (which is why follow up treatments exist), the fact remains that the underlying cause of the lower back pain has not been (and is not being) addressed, only its symptoms.

CAUSES OF LOWER BACK PAIN

QUESTION: What causes lower back pain?

ANSWER: There are many different causes of lower back pain. And there's been a lot of action taken in terms of treating degenerative disc disease and particularly herniated discs that are often a legitimate cause of lower back pain. The solution is typically surgery for most conditions of this nature, but the data on such conditions is not entirely conclusive. For instance, if one takes a hard look at the studies that have been conducted on herniated discs, what one finds is that when an MRI is performed on a cohort of patients that are both asymptomatic and symptomatic with lower back pain, the incidents of legitimate herniated discs is the same in both groups – but only one group experiences symptoms of pain. In other words, a lot of the times when one believes that a herniated disc is causing these symptoms, it's a case of "true," "maybe true" or "unrelated." In a lot of instances of lower back pain we don't know what is the real cause of the pain. For instance, is it muscular in nature? Have one of the deep lumbar muscles been strained or injured in some way? Is it a tendonitis? Is it an inflammation of the discs that sit between vertebrae? Is it actually coming from a herniated disc impinging on a nerve? We really can't pinpoint what the root cause is in most instances, and in most cases the lower back pain will self-correct irrespective of what modality one employs to relieve the symptoms – from massage all the way up to surgery. Knowing this phenomenon, one can well appreciate that what is known about lower backs is that: One, conditions that one would expect to cause considerable pain – such as degenerative and herniated discs – often do not produce any symptoms of pain in patients; and, two, most symptoms will go away on their own within anywhere from 24-hours to 12-weeks. And knowing this has unfortunately also allowed many people to ply their trade – whether that be chiropractic, massage therapy, trigger-point therapy, nerve root injections, fill in the blank – while Mother Nature simply takes her course, and then these people step in, take credit for the symptom relief -- and charge patients for the "service" they provided. It is in human nature to seek causation where causation may not exist, and a patient in pain (and who is unaware of the above facts) is particularly vulnerable and willing to return for such treatments since while receiving them his pain went away (which it would have done anyway, given the nature of the self-correction process).

LOWER BACK PAIN AND EVOLUTIONARY BIOLOGY

QUESTION: Why are humans so susceptible to lower back pain?

ANSWER: Our species is vulnerable to lower back pain largely because of our evolution from a knuckle-walking creature to an upright walking creature. This change in our posture, coupled with a very acute lordotic curve in the lower back when in an upright posture, creates a lot of compression in that area. In addition, a lot of movement around the lumbar spine is carried out by the spinal erector muscles, and if one is engaged in long periods of standing or working, those larger, more superficial muscles can become fatigued. As a consequence, a shifting of the workload takes place from the bigger, stronger spinal erector muscles onto the smaller and deeper multifidus muscles of the lower back that typically fatigue quicker than the spinal erector muscles (and, thus, are more vulnerable to injury). These deeper muscles are usually spared by the larger, more superficial muscles of the lower back, with the result that they can become relatively de-conditioned over time. Consequently, when the workload shifts from the lumbar muscles to these smaller and deeper muscles, they are more likely to become injured, strained or to spasm, thus resulting in considerable lower back pain. [1, 2]

THE MULTIFIDUS MUSCLES AND LOWER BACK RX

QUESTION: Was the ability to isolate and strengthen the multifidus muscles one of the main reasons why Arthur Jones had such success with his MedX Lumbar Spine Machine?

ANWER: Absolutely. The break through feature on the MedX Lumbar Spine machine was that, for the first time, a person could be restrained in this machine in such a way that any rotation around the hip joint was eliminated. As a result, any contribution from the buttock muscles and the more superficial lumbar muscles was eliminated, allowing one to effectively isolate the multifidus muscles and strengthen them. Jones was one of the first to really focus on this problem and conduct tests on the effects of direct exercise and rehabilitation. Some interesting data that came out of Jones' research was that he found that the frequency of applying the exercise stimulus in treating the lower back had to be far less than it is for other muscle groups in the body. The reason for this is that the MedX Lumbar Spine machine directed its focus to the multifidus muscles – not the spinal erector muscles. When most people think of the lower back musculature they envision the spinal erector muscles, which originate on the sacrum and the posterior iliac crest of the hip, and, crossing the hip joint, go up to the level of the thoracic vertebrae and the posterior ribs. Their function is to extend the entire torso. But because they cross the hip joint, they are one of the musculatures that produce rotation of the hip as one extends one's back. In order to target the deeper multifidus muscles, one must be placed in a position of mechanical insufficiency for the spinal erector muscles. That is, one's thighs, shins, and posterior hip need to be placed in a position where lumbar extension cannot contribute to the extension of back. Consequently, the load is shifted directly onto the multifidus muscles. When you look at the data that Jones' amassed in training these muscles, one notes that they fatigue rapidly and recover slowly, which is a profile very similar (if not identical) to fast-twitch muscle fibers. By contrast, the fatigue rate of the more superficial lumbar extensor musculature is slow but they possess a fast recovery ability, which is indicative of a slow-twitch muscle fiber profile. This makes sense, given that the spinal erectors are muscles of posture that are always active, don't produce huge amounts of force, are very slow to fatigue and quick to recover. Consequently, if one performs any sort of work that fatigues that musculature quickly enough, then the spinal erector muscles are going to seek support from the deeper musculature. And as a consequence of fatiguing quickly and recovering slowly, the optimal workout for strengthening the multifidus muscles would be extraordinarily brief – one set probably lasting less than 90-seconds– and performed very infrequently (perhaps once every 14-to-21-days).

CLOSE UP: THE MULTIFIDUS MUSCLES

QUESTION: I'm intrigued by what you've said about the Multifidus muscles (I've never heard of these before!)

Can you tell me more about them and their function?

ANSWER: The Multifidus are very small muscles that jump from one lumbar vertebrae to another. They extend at the top from the medial aspect of the transverse process of the spine, and they hop down to the next level attaching more laterally on the transverse process below. Their function is to connect one spinal segment to another, but all of those connections occur within the lumbar spine itself, not crossing the hip joint (ala the spinal erector muscles). The multifidus muscles produce lumbar extension but produce it at a single joint level between one vertebrae and the next. The various individual multifidus muscles possess the capacity to act in unison, creating a kind of kinetic chain that produces a summation of rotational forces. The multifidus between L-1 and L-2 produces a certain rotational force. And the multifidus between L-2 and L-3 also produces a certain rotational force – and so on for the multifidus muscles between L-3 and L-4 and L-4 and L-5 and so on. If the rotational angle is calculated for each section and one were to draw a straight line through the apex of that angle for each level what one will find is that a rotational point has been created that is actually outside the plane of the body and posterior to it – and this is the summation of all of the individual rotations of the many multifidus muscles. And this becomes the real genius of Jones' machine; i.e., that not only is one constrained in the machine so that the more superficial spinal erectors really can't contribute much to the movement because of mechanical insufficiency problems, but also if one looks at the rotational axis of the machine, one will find that the pivot point is to a certain distance posterior to the lumbar spine and exterior to the body. And what that rotation point actually ends up being is the summation point for all the different multifidi as they jump from one level to the next.

MULTIFIDUS LOWER BACK PAIN: A SCENARIO

QUESTION: Can you give me a scenario wherein one develops lower back pain as a result of straining his multifidus muscles? I want to see if perhaps this has been the same sort of situation that may have led to my lower back problem.

ANSWER: Sure. An individual is working in a warehouse. He has been on his feet for six hours straight and his spinal erector muscles are fatiguing over the course of the day. And as they fatigue – and remember they are larger, supporting shock-absorbing muscles that are fatiguing and are starting to drop out of the equation – his multifidus muscles pick up the slack. But their fatigue rate is a Fast Twitch profile and they fatigue rapidly. After his seventh hour of work, he drops his pen on the floor. He quickly bends down to pick it up when – Bam! – he suddenly feels a sharp, stabbing pain in his lower back that brings him to his knees. He'll be off work for an indefinite period of time with "some type of back problem." The sudden bending movement he made, resulted in a quick acceleration force being imposed upon his multifidus muscles that had up until this point been bearing the brunt of the workload and were becoming fatigued. It must be remembered that one of the primary functions of the surrounding supporting musculature (such as in the neck or lower back) is to become activated to protect your body in case of injury. For instance, if you fell off a cliff and upon hitting the ground fractured one of your lumbar vertebrae, the ligaments that connect one vertebral segment to another can become torn in that circumstance, with the result that you now have an acute injury to the lower back. Should this happen, the job of the deeper muscles such as the multifidus is to go into a very aggressive contraction to prevent any subluxation or movement of the lumbar vertebrae, which could result in a transection of your spinal cord or impingement of the nerve segments called the cauda equina (which is Latin for "Horse's tail," as it contains all of the lumbar/sacral nerves that come out off the base of the spinal cord) as any shifting of these fractured vertebrae could cause paralysis. Consequently, when someone is fatigued and then suffers an acute injury that produces pain, that pain produces a perception in the central nervous system that there has been an injury to the lower back and that, in turn, produces a reflex contraction of the multifidus muscles in that area to prevent any potential movement of a possible fracture that could threaten the spinal cord. Consequently, these deep muscles are very spasm-prone because they serve a protective function in the case of injury and acute pain can often produce a perception of injury that can activate this reflex-response.

LOWER BACK THERAPY

QUESTION: What would you recommend in terms of therapy for treating a lower back disorder brought about in such a way as you've described?

ANSWER: During the acute phase of a lower back injury, sometimes all one can really do is let Nature run its course, because once the multifidus muscles are contracting to protect the spine, it simply takes a certain amount of time for them to give up the contraction. Now this doesn't mean that one has to completely rest the injured area, because there is no solid scientific evidence that shows that bed rest or non-activity hastens the recovery process in such matters. Sometimes simply just carrying on with the normal activities of daily life (as best as one can under the circumstances) appears to be the best thing to do. In other words, during the acute phase the best remedy may be to simply wait it out until the pain starts to abate a little bit. And the thing that seems to give the signal for it to abate is just carrying out normal activities of daily life. Because if one has truly fractured one's lumbar spine, one is not going to be able to move or get about and inactivity and immobilization is a signal for a continuation of the protective/contraction process. By contrast, simply carrying out the normal activities of daily life sends a message of, "It seemed like we were pretty badly hurt at first, but now there's no evidence that there's a lumbar fracture that we have to continue this contraction process for." However, once one has gotten through the acute phase, where any movement at all is painful (and this can last anywhere from 72-hours to a week), then one is ready to start doing a range-of-motion-tolerable strengthening program. And make no mistake, this may temporarily exacerbate symptoms, but in the long run the strengthening that occurs is going to be protective to the musculature and prevent a similar injury (and its symptoms) from occurring in the future. After the acute phase, when one is ready to perform some strengthening exercise for the lower back and multifidus muscles, it would be ideal to seek out a MedX lumbar spine machine. However, these are rare and not many facilities have them (or the trained personnel that know how to operate them). If one cannot locate a center that has such a machine, a Nautilus lower back machine can be adapted in such a way as to emphasize or target the multifidus muscles. Even an overhead cable pulldown machine, if one is able to grip the bar with one's arms straight and one's legs under the roller pads, can be effective. The key in this movement is to consciously try to eliminate any hip rotation and, keeping the arms locked straight, simply perform a back extension, where one is consciously focusing on only activating the multifidus (deeper back) muscles. Such a movement can target those muscles quite successfully.

A NON-WEIGHTED MULTIFIDUS EXERCISE

One of the best things that I've found for activating the multifidus muscles is actually a form of non-weighted manual resistance taught to me by SuperSlow developer Ken Hutchins. Simply lie down on your back on the floor so that your hips and your shoulder blades are in contact with the floor. Now scrunch down so that your shoulder blades are pushed downward towards your hips – so you're shortening the distance between your shoulder blades and your hips. This produces a small arch in your back. Now what I want you to do is, very gradually, imagine pushing your shoulder blades and your hips into the floor and pushing your belly button out while you arch your back, trying to create as acute an arch as you can in your lumbar area by pushing your shoulder blades and your hips into the floor. Now gradually take the effort of that up to 25% and hold that 25% effort for 15-seconds. Slowly relax the contraction and then perform another contraction, this time taking the level of force up to 50% for 15-seconds. After easing off the contraction, pause for 10-seconds and then perform the movement again, this time at 75% of your maximum force. Again, push your belly button towards the ceiling and create more of an acute arch in your lumbar spine and sustain this contraction for 15-seconds. Now slowly release the contraction. Finally, take your force output up to 100% and hold it for 15-seconds. Now relax the contraction slowly. By performing this movement in this fashion you will have immobilized your pelvis by lying on the floor, and you will have immobilized your upper spine by pinning your shoulder blades to the floor. Creating that forceful arch in your back is actually the same arch that you get in Arthur's machine, and you've just performed a good Timed Static Contraction exercise for your multifidus. And now that you're up moving around again you can feel the same sort of burn and fatigue in the deep lumbar muscles that you feel when you get off Arthur's machine. That's how I perform a Timed Static Contraction with clients who are having low back problems to get at their multifidus without having a MedX machine. And if you want to progress this, you could place weights on your abdomen or even start with a phone book. It's best to do it by having a good partner or a good trainer provide manual resistance over the belly button as you're trying to push it up toward the ceiling – that will increase the effect. I would have someone perform this no more than once a week and better yet once every 14-days.

-- Doug McGuff, MD

When people come to the authors' facility with back problems we have them perform a Max Contraction on a Nautilus Lower Back machine, a back extension on the pulldown machine or the non-weighted exercise just described. We then build a basic workout routine around the lower back exercise with the understanding that improving one's general conditioning will go a long, long way towards helping the rehabilitation process. If someone is being rehabbed for an acute lower back injury, it is also important that the exercises performed are not solely focused on his lower back area, but also on general strengthening. It is evident that the stronger one becomes in terms of one's surrounding supporting musculature, especially the musculature of the back – running as it does all the way from the buttocks to the base of the skull – the better one will be protected. The entire spine articulates in such a way that it cannot handle much in the way of force without the assistance of its surrounding supporting musculature. By building a stronger musculature, the increased strength is going to be protective to the spine, but in addition the increased muscle mass from a mechanical, shock-absorbing capability, is going to provide additional protection for the spine. Consequently, a well-rounded strength training program is going to go a long way towards protecting the entire back – upper and lower. If someone is training once a week, he might include lower back deep muscle exercise every other workout (or once every 14-days).

WORKING WITH ACUTE PAIN

QUESTION: *I'm a personal trainer and one of my clients has acute lower back pain. How should I train him so that I don't aggravate his condition?*

ANSWER: When training a client who has acute lower back pain one must operate within the constraints of what the client is able to do at that time, and this may be relatively limited. Nevertheless, even if this proves to be a very limited range of motion that the trainee can operate within (even if it's a motionless Timed Static Contraction or Max Contraction in that area), anything that initiates some strengthening within the constraints of a tolerable range of motion is a step towards accelerating the rate of the client's recovery. However, as trainers we can't take credit for this (for reasons already indicated), but even starting the process of strengthening that area will at least make the recurrence of lower back pain much less likely. What we have found to be effective when dealing with any joint of the body that has a compromised range of motion due to injury is to initially – without any weight–determine what the client's comfortable range of motion is and then apply resistance *only* within that comfortable range of motion, and strengthen within that comfortable range of motion. Over time, as the client is strengthened within that comfortable range of motion, we find that the comfortable range of motion starts to expand in either direction. And as that client's strength continues to increase, his range of motion continues to expand until it's normal. And it's been our experience that if one applies strengthening throughout a client's comfortable range of motion, as his range of motion expands to normal he will also be strengthened well enough to protect against future bouts of dysfunction.

BLOOD FLOW AS CURATIVE

I have a theory that in some instances – and I've noted this whenever we've performed any type of rehabilitation involving lower backs – a lot of lower back problems are more often than not muscle related. As blood is the best healer there is (as it brings nutrients to the area to facilitate growth and repair of damaged tissue and it removes the waste products that accrue as a result of repair), what I've found is that anything that draws blood to the problem area is therapeutic. We use a Max Contraction for this purpose, which is a little bit like clamping off a garden hose; i.e., during the contraction blood flow to the area is constricted, but immediately upon cessation of the contraction blood surges into the area bringing with it an abundance of the nutrients necessary for repair. This tends to bring a lot of symptom relief. Moreover, it sometimes would appear that the problem (or impingement) is quite often the by-product of what I call a "rogue motor unit" that has engaged. And if you can increase blood flow to the afflicted area, doing so brings many nutrients, the most important in this instance being calcium. The influx of calcium into the sarcoplasmic reticulum serves to disengage the actin and myosin heads of the muscle fiber and create muscular relaxation. Once the calcium has shut off the ignition of that contraction that's occurring within the motor unit and causing impingement, you've shut off the problem right at its source. In addition, we've talked about the body's protective-contraction response to a perceived injury in and around the spine. This, I would submit, is what I'm referring to as a "rogue motor unit" that, will self engage in a non-productive and inappropriate protracted contraction. Now the floor exercise that Doug has prescribed, or training on a MedX Lumbar extension machine, not only provides strengthening of the muscles to aid in a long-term rehab, but in the more acute phase what this is also doing is creating a situation through the application of low force that produces enough fatigue in that rogue motor unit that it can no longer sustain its contraction and finally lets go of it. So I think that during the acute phase, that might be the big benefit; i.e., that you've fatigued that muscle to the point where it can't up the contraction or spasm that has been causing you such discomfort.

-- John Little

HERNIATED DISC PROBLEMS

QUESTION: What should a person do for rehabilitation if they have suffered a herniated disc?

ANSWER: A herniated disc is a condition that may require medical treatment. We say "may," because it depends upon whether or not the herniated disc is protruding (and thus producing a mechanical compression on the central spinal cord, or producing a mechanical compression on the peripheral nerves as they exit the spinal cord such as a lumbar nerve root). The disc serves as a shock absorber that sits between the vertebrae and is made of fibrous connective tissue. In the middle of the disc is a gelatinous material that has a shock-absorptive capability. Discs can be likened to connective tissue that is constructed like a jelly donut, with the jelly in the middle. A disc becomes herniated when it encounters a compressive force that pushes the internal gelatinous material outside of the disc; i.e., the fibrous ring has become somewhat decomposed and degenerated, and, as a consequence of its encounter with a compressive force, some of its jelly-like center has leaked out of the disc. Once it has leaked out, it can either retreat in a straight line backward into the disc, thus causing compression on the spinal cord, or it can move out laterally to either side of the disc and compress one of the nerve roots in the process. If one has a herniated disc and it is producing a compression such as we've just described, that is a medical problem (and a potential medical emergency) that needs to be addressed by a competent physician and may require surgery to correct. If one has acutely herniated a disc, one can develop lumbar pain as a consequence, but this will resolve over time if there isn't nerve compression occurring and can be improved with proper strength training exercise. If one strengthens the musculature around a diseased disc then that stronger musculature will be better able to provide support for the disc and also provide a shock absorber effect of being able to absorb forces that would otherwise be passed on to the deranged disc. However, a herniated disc that does not cause compression is not a medical emergency and, in fact, is a condition that is as prevalent in asymptomatic people as it is in symptomatic people.

TENDONITIS

QUESTION: What is tendonitis? Can one rehabilitate this condition through resistance exercise?

ANSWER: Tendonitis is an injury that typically results from overuse of a particular tendon. For instance, a job that requires an individual to scan products at the checkout of a grocery store may find that the motion involved with scanning bar codes thousands of times per week can wear on the tendon on the radial aspect of the wrist and a tendonitis can develop. The suffix "itis" refers to inflammation, and tendonitis refers to a condition whereby both the tendon and the sheath that it slides through (in a manner very much like a stick going through a corn dog) both become inflamed. The therapy for tendonitis is always rest, as subjecting the tendon and its sheath to more of the repetitive movement that caused the inflammation will only make the condition worse and prolong the repair and recovery period. If the pain from the inflammation is severe, then a physician-prescribed course of non-steroidal or steroidal anti-inflammatory medicine for a period of five days will usually resolve it.

TENDONITIS VERSUS TENDONOPATHY

QUESTION: I've had really bad tendonitis for several years. I'm 35-years old and the problem just isn't going away. Any thoughts on why it has hung on for so long?

ANSWER: In some cases, particularly for those in their late thirties to early fifties, what is perceived as being a tendonitis is actually a tendonopathy. Years of overusing muscles (and consequently, the tendons that anchor muscles to bones) can develop a chronic pathology that is largely unaffected by anti-inflammatory medicines. Interestingly, the best treatment for tendonopathy is strength training, which strengthens both muscles and tendons, and, thus, enlarges the size of the muscles, which, in turn enlarges the shock-absorbing capacity of the muscles, which serves to dissipate the trauma that would otherwise be passed on to the tendonopathy. In most cases, making the muscles stronger will resolve the problem. However, this being true, it is also true that even though such a condition is not an "itis" (i.e., an inflammation), repetitive over use can still bring the tendonopathy to the point where it becomes symptomatic. Consequently, if one engages in an activity where one is chronically extending the wrist (in the case of forearm tendonopathies), such an activity will only serve to aggravate the tendonopathy. However, a program of progressive strengthening exercises can certainly protect one from having the tendonopathy coming to bear in one's activities of daily life. In cases such as the one indicated above, including direct exercise for the forearm muscles (such as those indicated in Chapter 10 of *Body By Science*) every two weeks (or every other workout) for the purpose of strengthening the forearm musculature will help resolve the problems encountered with tendonopathy.

ELBOWS – "GOLFER'S" AND "TENNIS"

QUESTION: How would you rehab someone with "golfer's elbow" and/or "tennis elbow" conditions?

ANSWER: A similar rehabilitative prescription would also apply to treating the inflammatory conditions of "golfer's elbow" and "tennis elbow." "Tennis elbow" is simply a lateral epicondylitis, or inflammation, at the point where the tendon of the extensor carpi radialis muscle inserts. "Golfer's elbow" is a medial epicondylitis, or an inflammation on the little bump on the inside aspect of one's elbow, where the tendon of the flexor carpi ulnaris inserts. Since both conditions are legitimate examples of an "itis," their rehabilitative treatments should be the same as they would be for any other cases of acute inflammation (i.e., a period of rest and perhaps non-steroidals for five days followed by strength training for the musculature containing the inflamed tendon).

TREATING ACUTE TENDONITIS

During periods of acute tendonitis (that is, in cases were the inflammation is chronic) one should allow a period of time to pass until one can at least perform one's strengthening/rehabilitative exercises without significantly exacerbating the pain symptoms. Since many patients that develop tendonitis will be placed on a course of steroid medication (typically synthetic corticosteroid drugs such as Prednisone) in an effort to resolve the inflammation, it's very important that one be careful not to perform rehabilitative strengthening exercise during this period of time, particularly if there is a chance that the tendonitis might actually be a tendonopathy. The reason being that when one is taking steroid medication, it decreases inflammation but can worsen the tendonopathy, making the inflamed tendon weaker and thus more prone to rupture. Consequently, if an individual has been placed on a course of steroids for tendonitis, he should hold off on his strength training exercises until he has been off of the drugs for a period of several days so that the exercise and anti-inflammatories don't weaken the tendon further.

-- Doug McGuff, MD

Once the patient has become asymptomatic the "Big 5" program outlined in Chapter 4 of *Body By Science* should be employed as it will go a long way in strengthening the muscles and tendons of the body. In other words, you don't always require *direct* work on the musculo-tendinous unit that has become inflamed in order to protect yourself from future flare ups. A more basic routine may involve enough work to strengthen

79

those muscles and their tendons to the point where they will never become symptomatic. But if it becomes acutely symptomatic, once you can get over the acute phase, performing some direct work that focuses on the area in question would certainly help. In the case of a "Tennis Elbow" condition, performing direct work on the musculatures involved in flexing and extending the wrist will serve to strengthen them and prove to be protective from the tendonitis condition re-occurring.

CHONDROMALACIA

QUESTION: One of my friends is a runner and she says she has a condition called "Chondrolmalacia." All I know is that she has a sore patella. What exactly is this condition?

ANSWER: Chondromalacia Patella is another common injury, involving the loss of articular cartilage on the underside of the patella. In the rehabilitation of such a condition, two factors become exceedingly important; one, again, the strengthening of the surrounding supporting musculature will prove to be very helpful, and, two, the person that is suffering this condition does not have Patellofemoral Syndrome (PFS). When looking at the kneecap from what is called a "sunrise view" (i.e., from the front), the patella forms a triangle shape. The patella rides on a groove on the distal femur where it fits perfectly into that groove, which becomes a track upon which the patella slides back and forth as the knee flexes and extends. If one has a balanced development of one's quadriceps musculature, the patella will always stay upon that track. However, in certain cases a muscular imbalance of the quadriceps muscles can cause the patella to jump the track, and this is where problems can arise. It is not uncommon for females (who genetically have a wider carrying angle at the hip) to have a relatively underdeveloped vastus medialis muscle (the "tear drop" shape muscle that resides on the medial aspect of the quadriceps), with the result that they experience a stronger pulling force from the lateral aspect of their quadriceps than they do from the medial aspect. This causes the patella to track laterally, in effect jumping the track that it normally would ride upon and can thus produce inflammation on the underside of the patella and on the patella tendon, owing to the fact that the patella is now attempting to track laterally and jump its track. In some instances if one contracts one's quadriceps with sufficient force (such as when one takes a forceful step or lands too hard from a jump) it can cause one's quadriceps to contract suddenly and violently, with the result that one can dislocate one's kneecap laterally. The proper treatment (both in a preventative sense and post trauma) for this condition is to have the patient strengthen the medial aspect of his quadriceps by performing exercises such as the Leg Extension, that allow him to isolate the last 15-degrees of extension, as this is the range in which the vastus medialis muscle of the quadriceps comes most strongly into play. An alternative strengthening exercise would be the Leg Press with an emphasis on fatiguing the musculature in the extended portion of its range of motion (where the leg is almost fully extended) as, again, this ensures that the vastus medialis muscle receives adequate stimulation to become stronger. It would not be advisable to perform both of these exercises in any given workout as that could represent too much work for an individual's recovery ability to overcome in seven-days time. It would be better to alternate performance of the two exercises from one workout to the next. Such exercises will serve to ensure that the muscular pulling force of the quadriceps will be increased on the medial side to bring it more in line with the pulling force that is operating from the lateral side, thus causing the patella to "get back on track," so to speak. Most patellar tendonitis is due to this lack of development on the medial quadriceps and the pulling of the patella in a lateral direction. Consequently, the use of single axis exercises (isolation exercises) can prove very helpful for purposes of rehabilitation, allowing one to target and strengthen problem areas.

ROTATOR CUFF

QUESTION: As a personal trainer I see a lot of people come into our facility complaining of having injured their "rotator cuff." What is a rotator cuff?

ANSWER: Interestingly, the term "rotator cuff" is a relatively recent one. You will not, for instance, find the term in *Gray's Anatomy*. It is more of a slang term that has found its way into the general parlance of rehabilitation. The shoulder joint is a ball and socket joint that is hyper mobile. Your shoulder has such an exquisitely huge range of motion that you can rotate it in any direction. But what you sacrifice for having this phenomenal range of motion is joint stability. The body has two ball and socket joints, located at the hip joint and shoulder. The hip joint accommodates the head of the femur, which has a relatively compact ball that is small. This ball is contained within a large socket that is big and therefore encompasses most of the ball. By contrast, the shoulder joint accommodates the head of the humerus, which has a very large ball that articulates with a very small socket. The actual size of the socket that this ball articulates within is approximately 10-to-15 percent of the articular surface. Consequently, there is nothing that is holding the ball in that socket apart from the surrounding musculature. To better understand the working of this joint, take the thumb and first three fingers of your right hand and imagine grabbing a billiard ball and pulling it into the palm of your hand such that your index finger and thumb come together. Instead of fingers, however, the body employs four tendons of the surrounding musculature, and instead of a billiard ball, they are grabbing onto the outer edge of the ball at the top of the humerus. The rotator cuff, then, is trying to hold this ball in the socket throughout this very large and wide range of motion. Now if you're holding that billiard ball in your right hand, take your left hand and cup it over the top of your right hand that is holding the ball. Your left hand represents the bone that comes off the shoulder blade (called the acromian process) and attaches to your collarbone, producing a boney roof over the ball and socket. However, as you take those four digits that are holding that billiard ball and rotate them around, you'll find that your fingers (representing the tendons coming into the shoulder) scrub against the roof of that ball and socket joint. In most cases what occurs with rotator cuff problems is that those tendons are operating within a very tight space underneath that boney roof, and because of certain types of movements and the forces involved, they end up scrubbing against the boney roof, and this is what causes inflammation to develop. In other situations they can be placed in a mechanical position (such as when throwing a baseball) that acutely overwhelm the ability of the tendons to hold the ball and socket together. Consequently, one can develop a tear in the rotator cuff tendons, particularly if one's arm is externally rotated and abducted too forcefully (or internally rotated and adducted too forcefully, as in the motion of trying to touch one's thumb between one's shoulder blades when one's arm is behind one's back). So if the range of motion becomes too extreme the strength of those tendons can become exceeded and they will tear. More commonly, one will perform a type of movement repetitively that chronically scrubs those tendons underneath that tight acromian joint and this can lead to long-term injury. So rotator cuff injuries are typically the result of shear forces on the tendons that occur repetitively over time until inflammation is initiated.

THE MUSCLES OF
THE "ROTATOR CUFF"

QUESTION: Are there muscles in the rotator cuff?

ANSWER: No, but there are muscles that attach to the tendons that make up the rotator cuff. If one looks at the shoulder blade, one will note that it appears to have a "spine" on it, and the position of the tendons relative to this spine represent the "SITS" component of the names of the muscles that these tendons attach to. And the tendons of the rotator cuff connect to four separate muscles; the supraspinatus ("supra" meaning "above" or "on top of" the shoulder blade, and, thus, above its spine); the infraspinatus ("infra" meaning that it is superficial on the shoulder blade and below its spine); the teres minor (which runs from the side of the shoulder blade and under the arm pit); and the supscapularis (which emanates from beneath the shoulder blade). And the tendons from these four muscles converge into the shoulder joint and attach to the ball of the humerus. Two of these tendons rotate externally, and two of them rotate internally, and, collectively, they make up what is popularly referred to as the "rotator cuff."

TREATING ROTATOR CUFF INJURY

QUESTION: *How would recommend one rehabilitate a client that has suffered an injury to his rotator cuff?*

ANSWER: If one develops an acute tendonitis in one or more of the tendons that make up the rotator cuff, the first thing that needs to happen – as with all tendonitis – is that it (or they) be rested in order to allow the inflammation to diminish. If there is not a specific tear that needs to be repaired, specific strengthening exercises can then be performed to strengthen the injured muscle/s and tendon/s. The following paragraphs describe manual resistance exercise for the rotator cuff developed by Ken Hutchins:

> If strengthening is performed to strengthen the muscles and tendons responsible for external rotation, the patient's upper arm should be pulled in tight against the side of his torso and manual resistance should be applied by the trainer to the patient's wrist as he attempts external rotation to the greatest range he is capable of. The patient will note that when his hand is closest to his abdomen (at the beginning of the movement) he can produce a considerable amount of force, but as he continues the external rotation his force output will drop off markedly, requiring (and tolerating) very little in the way of counter force on the part of the one applying the manual resistance.

> If exercise is to be performed for the purpose of strengthening the muscles and tendons responsible for internal rotation, the patient should, again, begin the movement with his upper arm pinned into the side of his torso (and the trainer, again, resisting manually), but this time starting from a position of external rotation where his forearm moves from an outward to an inward position.

Both of these movements should be performed as a series of repetitions in a progressive fashion in terms of the patient's force output. For instance, during the first repetition the patient should be producing approximately 25 percent of his potential force as the trainer resists the movement. The second repetition will require that he bring his force output up to roughly 50 percent. The third repetition should be performed at 75 percent of the patient's strength, while the fourth and final repetition should be performed at 100 percent of the patient's strength. The repetitions should be performed slowly so that the patient is moving his limb at approximately a 10-seconds out and 10-seconds back cadence. As the one applying the manual resistance, the trainer will discover that the patient is actually stronger during the first repetition he performs (the one requiring 25 percent of the patient's strength) than he is during the last repetition (the one requiring 100 percent of his strength) owing to the fatigue that the patient has accumulated by this point, which will cause his strength to diminish markedly.

These two exercises would be all that we would recommend for rehabilitating the tendons of the rotator cuff.

THE IMPORTANCE OF BUILDING STRENGTH IN THE SURROUNDING MUSCULATURE

QUESTION: Once the symptoms have improved, would it benefit the individual who has suffered an injury to the rotator cuff to then move on to perform the "Big 5" workout as indicated in Body By Science?

ANSWER: The upper body exercises in the "Big 5" workout will serve to provide strengthening for the surrounding muscles that support the shoulder joint, such as the pectoralis, trapezius, latissimus dorsi, and the rhomboids. All of these muscle groups contribute to the well being of the shoulder joint by providing both a protective shock-absorptive capability and strength.

These exercises have been placed in the "Big 5" workout for three reasons; one, they track muscle and joint function properly, thus reducing wear and tear issues; two, they involve the greatest amount of muscle groups in their performance, thus providing stimulation to all of the major muscle groups of the body; and, three, they not only effectively load the musculature but, in the case of the Pulldown and Overhead Press, do so in a way that doesn't close up the acromian space and produce an impingement problem. For instance, if instead of a close-grip, palms-up pulldown we had recommended that the trainee perform a wide-grip, palms-down pulldown behind the neck (a common version of the pulldown exercise that is performed in many gymnasiums around the world) then his arms would be abducted away from his body and the upper arm would be externally rotated away from his shoulder. The result would be that he would be loading the upper back musculatures and producing a movement that could cause impingement as a result of the way he would have positioned his humerus within the shoulder joint. Whenever one is performing an exercise that requires the arms to be placed above one's head -- whether it be a type of pulldown or an overhead press – it is important that one's hands stay in a plane that is visible to the eye (in one's peripheral vision). Doing so will ensure that one is in a mechanical position that is not going to produce impingement of the shoulder. By contrast, if one is producing movement in an overhead plane in such a fashion that the hands are no longer visible in one's peripheral vision, the chances of impinging the shoulder joint are dramatically increased.

REHAB FREQUENCY FOR THE ROTATOR CUFF

QUESTION: You had mentioned that the lower back muscles don't need to be trained for rehabilitation as often as other skeletal muscles. Would the same recommendation hold true for training the rotator cuff area?

ANWER: No, unlike the lower back, one may benefit

from performing the specific rehabilitation exercises for the rotator cuff a little more frequently than once every two weeks (or every other workout). The manually resisted exercises indicated can be performed every workout (or once a week) and in concert with the regular "Big 5" routine outlined in Chapter 4 of *Body By Science*. During the acute phase of rotator cuff rehab, where re-establishing the client's range of motion is a priority, one may be able to perform these exercises perhaps twice a week without ill consequence.

THE PROBLEM WITH RUBBER BANDS

An interesting thing about typical rehabilitation approaches is that physiotherapists are quite fond of using a rubber (also known as surgical) tubing apparatus to perform movements similar to what we have outlined. However, if you perform the manual resistance rotator cuff exercises as we've described, what you'll find is that when the client is performing an external rotation his force at the beginning of the movement is quite high and the force that he is able to provide when he's fully externally rotated is quite low. And the opposite, of course, is true with internal rotation; it starts out relatively high and then drops again. Consequently, what you'll find if you're using rubber tubing for rehab is that the strength curve is exactly backwards from what it needs to be; i.e., when the force output from the subject is high, the rubber tubing is not yet stretched, so the force it supplies is quite low; when the subject achieves full external rotation that is when his force output is the weakest, but that's when he's fully stretching the rubber band and its force output is the highest. So if you're using rubber tubing as your therapeutic modality the strength curve is entirely backwards for the movement that you're trying to do. So that's why we prefer using manual resistance, as the trainer can provide a perfect match to the subject's strength curve in both internal and external rotation movements.

-- Doug McGuff, MD

PULLED GROIN MUSCLES

QUESTION: I keep hearing on TV about athletes suffering from a "pulled groin muscle." What is this condition exactly?

ANSWER: In most instances a pulled groin muscle is the result of an acute high force injury. The best thing one can do to heal or rehabilitate such an injury is to simply allow the injured muscle and/or its tendon sufficient time to recover. If the individual who has suffered a pulled groin muscle is involved in a sport that's obviously made that area vulnerable, then once the acute inflammatory phase has passed, he or she should perform either direct strength training exercise for the hip adductors (which can be done on either a Nautilus or MedX machine) or manual resistance exercise for these muscles. The latter exercise should be performed with the subject lying on the floor and the trainer applying manual resistance for adduction (or abduction if necessary) with the same 25 percent, 50 percent, 75 percent, and 100 percent pattern that we employed with the lower back and rotator cuff exercises. However, such exercises should only be required if strengthening actually needs to be performed for this area owing to an inherent weakness in this muscle group or the fact that the subject is involved in a high force sport where further acute high force trauma is likely to re-occur. If the groin pull was the result of just a fluke occurrence (such as a slip or fall), then all that's required is a chance for the adductor muscle (or muscles, if both legs are afflicted) to recover. At which point simply starting or resuming a basic strength-training program is usually sufficient to prevent such an injury from occurring again.

REHAB FOR KNEE INJURIES

QUESTION: As a strength and conditioning coach I've seen all manner of knee injuries -- ligamentous injuries such as a torn meniscus, torn collateral ligaments, and most commonly, torn cruciate ligaments that require specialized rehabilitation. If someone has to have surgery to repair a torn cruciate ligament, for instance, how should one go about restoring range of motion and exercising the area?

ANSWER: This will depend upon the modality used

during surgery and what type of materials were used. For instance, did the surgeon use a cadaveric graft? Did he use a graft off a person's own tendon from elsewhere on the body? Did he employ a synthetic graft? These are relevant issues facing a rehabilitation specialist as the answers to these questions factor into what the tolerance of these various graphs are, and how much active force needs to be applied to reestablish the patient's range of motion. If it's a post-operative ligamentous derangement of the knee, it is best to leave the rehabilitation to specialists in this field, for the simple fact that the authors have limited knowledge of these specialized surgical procedures and their immediate post-operative effects. However, having said this, once the acute phase is over, strengthening the muscles that surround and support the knee is the best therapy. The acute phase in knee rehabilitation occurs after operative repair. Most times, however, after someone has undergone surgery resulting from a torn Anterior Cruiciate Ligament (ACL) and they have come out of a cast, the physiotherapists will attempt to perform some manual resistance to try and preserve the knee's range of motion, but they can often be overzealous in attempting to "force" range of motion into the injured joint. Clearly some of the rehabilitation modalities that we've seen are questionable. We've seen physiotherapists forcefully and manually apply resistance to a weakened joint in such a manner that there is no objective feedback on the forces being administered. A lot of physiotherapists also prescribe stretching to "strengthen" an injured joint or muscle, which such a modality simply can't achieve for reasons we've already covered elsewhere in both *Body By Science* and this book.

THE PROBLEM WITH LEG EXTENSIONS FOR REHAB

QUESTION: A lot of the rehab that is being done, particularly for cruciate ligament repairs, involves the use of a Leg Extension machine such as Cybex. Is this a good idea?

ANSWER: This can be a dubious choice of resistance exercise for this purpose for the simple fact that when the knee goes into full extension, the cruciate ligaments intertwine to some degree in what is called a "screw home" fashion. This involves the anterior and posterior cruciate ligaments wrapping over each other in a fashion not unlike wringing out a dishrag. Such a movement actually produces very high forces on the cruciate ligaments. This is not to suggest that all Leg Extension machines are dangerous or that they can't be helpful in rehabilitating the knee, but some leg extension machines (and unfortunately the ones that seem most prevalent in rehabilitation centers) are simply counterproductive for rehabilitative purposes.

THE MECHANICS OF AN EFFECTIVE LEG EXTENSION MACHINE

The only truly good Leg Extension machine that I've seen for rehabilitative purposes was one that was designed by Ken Hutchens, which is very much like a MedX Leg Extension but with a sliding platform that allows a little fore and aft sliding as the person performs the extension. This is important because the pivot point at the knee is not actually a single rotational axis; if you look at the end of the femur bone it has an offset "C" shaped curve to it along which the tibia slides. So it's not a *single rotational* axis, it's actually a *sliding* axis. And if you load the knee on a machine that has a fixed axis, and you go into full extension, the forces of that screw home function of the cruciate ligaments is greatly magnified, particularly if there's not an appropriate fall off in extension like the University of Florida norms say there needs to be. If you look at the University of Florida norms on the MedX machine for knee extension you'll see that there is a gradual rise in the force output until you one gets to a position of full extension, at which point there is a precipitous fall off to below baseline levels. Most Leg Extension machines load in such a fashion that they get heaviest at this point, rather than precipitously lighter, with the result that you have a combination of many factors that are problematic; i.e., a single rotational axis, the screw home function of the cruciate ligaments, and a strength curve that loads up instead of dropping off, and those three things converge to

put a really high force on a vulnerable area. So I've always had a theoretical problem with the way a lot of rehab has been done for the cruciate ligaments when it involves the use of a typical Leg Extension machine. And while I've got to admit that there's not a lot of bodies piling up and people who have ruptured their grafts by using typical Leg Extension machines in their rehab, just because you've been able to get away with something doesn't necessarily mean it's the right thing to do. I think that there are solid theoretical reasons as to why knee extensions, performed in the manner that they have been in most rehab environments (which is mostly with a Cybex machine on a single rotational axis that loads up heavy at the end of extension), could be harmful.
-- **Doug McGuff, MD**

And while the post-operative strengthening of the musculature surrounding and supporting the knee joint is the right thing to do, the Leg Extension (particularly of the single-joint axis variety), might pose more problems than it resolves. A Leg Press machine would be a far better exercise for the subject to employ, particularly if it is later generation Nautilus or MedX leg press, or a machine that has movement that is on a 4-bar linkage. A sled-like leg press can be potentially dangerous because there is no movement around both the hip and knee joints, such as occurs with a MedX leg press. With a sled style leg press there is a lot more rotation around the knee joint than there is around the hip joint, with the result that at the point of full flexion there is a lot of sheer force produced in the knee. By contrast, with a Nautilus or MedX leg press, there is movement through a 4-bar linkage in such a manner that foot plate is not only moving straight out from the subject, but it's also moving out and down simultaneously, thus providing at least as much rotation in the hip as there is in the knee. This makes it not only an effective strengthening exercise for the muscles that support and serve the knee joint, but also a very protective exercise. The Leg Press exercise, as part of an overall strength-training program performed once a week, will prove to be a very effective rehabilitation for injured knees. It might be necessary to reduce the range of motion initially (along the lines of what we suggest with arthritic subjects) to a range that is comfortable for the subject, but over time the subject's range will increase with strengthening and, unlike some other rehabilitation modalities for the knee, it will do so without enhancing the chance of increased sheer force into the knee joint.

BURSITIS

QUESTION: When I was younger, my father always used to complain about suffering from "bursitis." What is this condition and could he have used strength training to treat it?

ANSWER: We don't hear as much about bursitis as we hear about other injuries, but bursitis is a more common affliction than one might suspect. A bursa is a fluid filled sack that is situated at a joint over a boney prominence. Its function is to serve as a shock absorber for joints. For instance, overlying the greater trochanter of the hip is the trochanteric bursa, and just underneath the kneecap is the prepatellar bursa. Both of these serve as shock absorbers for where the tendons move over a joint. And a lot of times a bursitis will occur because of direct pressure or direct trauma to the area overlying that bursa, such as when one suffers a direct contact injury to the iliac greater trochanter of the femur, (also known as a "hip pointer") such as might occur after one received a punishing hit to the lateral aspect of the hip, such as occurs in sports like hockey and football. However, other times a bursitis can occur due to wear and tear as a result of repetitive motion activities, such as the recurrent trauma that occurs in marathon runners when the iliotibial band constantly rubs over the lateral femoral epicondyle, which, when combined with the repeated flexion and extension of the knee during running, often causes the area to become inflamed. Other times a bursitis can develop as a result of jobs or activities that require one to work while kneeling (resulting in a prepatellar bursitis). A trochanteric bursitis can occur from either a direct trauma, such as getting hit by a hockey or football player's helmet, or by the athlete falling and landing hard on his hip. The way that most bursitis conditions are resolved is through resting the injured area and (occasionally) with anti-inflammatory medication. Typically, however, simply resting the area from the activity that has caused the inflammation will take care of the problem. After rest, strengthening the musculature can prove very helpful, as if one develops a stronger, wider muscle belly to serve a shock absorptive capability it will spare the bursa to a large measure. The "Big 5" workout indicated in Chapter 4 of *Body By Science* will prove helpful in this respect.

NECK PAIN

QUESTION: I enjoyed your chapter on Athletics in Body By Science *and was impressed at the need for strengthening the neck. Given how important this is, I'm curious as to why there is no direct neck work in the "Big 5" workout and also if using direct neck work might help to alleviate neck pain issues?*

ANSWER: Neck training is a beneficial thing for most people to do – whether they play a sport or not. We did not include direct neck work in with our "Big 5" workout as exercises such as the Seated Row, Pulldown and Overhead Press help will involve muscles such as the trapezius, which are supportive of the neck. However, if you train at a professional facility that has a good neck machine (such as those made by Nautilus and MedX), then we would strongly recommend that you use it. Even if you're not having any neck problems, even if you're not a football player or a hockey player or a wrestler, it will still behoove you to train your neck every other workout (or once every two weeks) as it will prove to be a very potent form of preventative medicine. After all, no one can predict when they might be rear-ended in a traffic accident and, should that happen, having a strong surrounding neck musculature, particularly the larger more superficial muscles of the neck, will go a long way towards protecting those deeper structures.

ANTI-WHIPLASH MEDICINE

I was rear ended in a car accident several months prior to the writing of *Body By Science* and to this day

I haven't felt a thing – as opposed to many people who come into Emergency Rooms of various hospitals after a similar experience and present with significant whiplash syndrome because of the fact that they have a 15-pound head sitting on a spindly weak neck.

-- Doug McGuff, MD

As indicated above, a lot of trainees will develop a very strong neck simply as a result of performing the "Big 5" program that we outlined in Chapter 4. This occurs from what is popularly referred to as the "indirect effect" of exercise (the fact that stimulation of the larger muscle groups of the body has a carry over effect, whereby the smaller muscle groups also receive stimulation, albeit to a slightly lesser degree), as well as the involvement of the neck in stabilization during heavy work. Nevertheless, we believe that direct neck work, particularly when a qualified trainer oversees it, can prove to be extraordinarily beneficial. And a lot of times neck problems occur simply because the surrounding supporting musculature is weak. And these are symptoms that can easily be relieved by improving the strength of the surrounding supporting musculature of the neck.

POST-CORONARY REHABILITATION

QUESTION: I recently suffered a heart attack. I want to start strength training but my cardiologist recommends against it and wants me to do "cardio" on a treadmill. What are your thoughts?

ANSWER: The profound effect of resistance training on the cardiovascular system might make one worry that the demands are too great and resistance training may actually be dangerous to those with known or lurking cardiovascular disease. However, an understanding of how your cardiovascular system works, coupled with a review of the scientific literature reveals that such worries are unfounded. When most people speak of "doing cardio," the "cardio" they are referring to is the cardiovascular system. The function of your cardiovascular system is to pump oxygen and nutrient rich blood to the tissues of your body. The "cardio" in cardiovascular refers to your heart. Your heart's contribution is its pumping action that moves the blood through your body. The "vascular" in cardiovascular refers to your blood vessels, which include the arterial system that carries blood from your heart to your organs and the venous system which carries blood back from your organs to your heart. Your blood vessels can change their caliber and thus affect the resistance that your heart has to pump against, which in turn affects how much blood can be pushed forward with each beat of your heart. Your heart produces blood flow or *cardiac output* through its heart rate and its stroke volume (how much blood pushed forward per heartbeat). If you need to increase your cardiac output, you can do so by increasing your heart rate, increasing your stroke volume or both. You can also increase your cardiac output by dilating the arteries and decreasing the resistance (called *peripheral vascular resistance*) that the heart must pump against. One last way to increase cardiac output is to increase the amount of blood returning to your heart. Your heart functions much like a sump pump, in the sense that whatever volume is brought into the pump is the volume that is pushed out of the pump. Thus, if you increase the amount of blood returning to the heart from the venous side of the circulation, you will increase the amount of blood pumped out of the heart (in physiology circles this is known as *Starling's Law of the Heart*). With a basic understanding of cardiovascular physiology one can now see the various ways that one may enhance one's cardiovascular functioning by increasing one's cardiac output. One can strengthen one's heart so that it pumps more with each beat (increased stroke volume). One can increase one's heart rate in times of demand. One can have more plentiful and more pliable blood vessels so that one's heart has to pump against less resistance (lower systemic vascular resistance-lower blood pressure). Or one can enhance venous return to the heart. Traditional aerobic exercise has been known to produce many of these positive adaptations. Most of this has been demonstrated using a test called a V02max, which is a measure of oxygen utilization during exercise. Scientists have found that

VO2max tracks cardiac output and have thus used it as an indirect measure of how effectively a particular exercise is at stimulating the cardiovascular system. The use of this test is one of the main reasons that resistance training was at one point believed to be a poor stimulator of the cardiovascular system. It seems that at the very high levels of exertion seen in resistance training VO2max falls off. Rather than assuming something may be flawed with the test, however, most scientists assumed that cardiac output must fall during weight training. They reasoned that the contracting and engorged muscles squeezed the blood vessels and increased peripheral vascular resistance and trapped venous blood, which then inhibited cardiac return. In addition to decreasing cardiac output, many believed that resistance training dangerously raised blood pressure (despite maintaining that it had little effect on the heart). As a consequence, most "authorities" claimed that resistance training was unsafe for those with heart disease because it placed too great a strain on the heart. A basic understanding of the cardiovascular system, however, reveals the exact opposite; i.e., that resistance training has a profoundly positive effect on the cardiovascular system. The reason the muscles pump up and become engorged is directly due to increased blood flow from increased cardiac output. When you perform intense muscular exercise, adrenaline causes the arteries in your gut to constrict and the arteries in your muscles to dilate. This diverts blood flow to your working muscles (and is why your Mom told you not to swim right after eating). The dilation of these arteries causes a decrease in peripheral vascular resistance, which allows an increase in cardiac output. Furthermore, the "pump" that occurs in the muscles along with the squeezing actions of the working muscles actually "milks" blood from the venous system back towards the heart. Veins, unlike arteries, have very little tone; they serve as passive conduits of blood. The major way that blood in the veins is made to move back towards the heart is by the milking action of the working muscles. Consequently, the more intensely a muscle is made to contract, the more profound will be this milking action. This increased blood return to the heart creates a need for an increased cardiac output because of Starling's Law of the Heart. Even more important is the fact that coronary artery blood flow is dependent on blood return to the heart, which increases the blood leaving the aorta. As blood leaves the aorta it rushes forward. During diastole (the relaxation phase of the heartbeat) aortic blood washes back into the coronary arteries. An increase in cardiac output as a result of increased venous return causes a rise in the *end diastolic blood flow* in the aorta, and coronary artery blood flow is proportionate to end diastolic blood flow. We mention this because of observations we have made in many of our clients. We have some clients with known coronary artery narrowing, and this coronary artery disease causes them to have *angina*, which is heart pain due to poor coronary artery blood flow. Despite exercising these subjects at a relatively high level of intensity, we have never had any episodes of angina. These same clients, however, will experience angina when walking uphill or exercising on a treadmill or cycling on a stationary bike.

THE PROBLEM WITH WALKING

I don't believe that activities such as walking produce intense enough muscular contractions to stimulate increased venous return, which would augment end diastolic blood flow and coronary artery bloodflow. I believe resistance training increases venous return and coronary blood flow so that these subjects can tolerate a much higher intensity of exercise without experiencing angina. Despite many experts' concern that resistance training may not be safe for those with coronary artery disease, I believe we may come to find that it is the only form of exercise safe for these people. Furthermore, since steady state exercise increases demands on the heart without a significant enhancement of venous return and coronary blood flow, it may be the most dangerous form of exercise for cardiac rehab patients. Currently, most cardiac rehab programs emphasize the development of "aerobic conditioning" before any resistance training is considered. In the future, I believe we should not consider exposing these people to aerobic exercise until they have developed an adequate base of strength conditioning through proper resistance training.

Doug Mcguff, MD

To better understand why this is so, we need to review both the information and the illustrations that we presented in *Body By Science* in our chapter on Global Metabolic Conditioning. What's happened in both the fitness and rehabilitation worlds is that there has been such a long tradition that followed Dr. Kenneth Cooper's mintage of the word "aerobics" (particularly the aerobics craze that resulted from his best-selling books and that has endured now for over 40-years) that the general populace has taken it as almost being self-evident that the aerobic subsystem of metabolism is (somehow) directly linked to our species' cardiovascular health. The medical/scientific reality, however, is that the aerobic element is simply a specific metabolic aspect of adaptation that takes place within the entirety of any given cell within the body. In other words, the cardiovascular system serves the functioning of the entire cell – and not simply one aspect of it (such as the aerobic metabolic pathways). Indeed, one can make other specific metabolic adaptations that involve the entire cell that are not aerobic but that are also served by the cardiovascular system. As we've indicated before, it is the muscles that are the windows to the body and its state of health. All of these metabolic adaptations that we think are cardiovascular are not; there is no central cardiovascular adaptation, per se. One may have measurable changes in cardiovascular parameters, but these are a direct result of specific metabolic adaptations that occur in the periphery (i.e., in the muscle). And the idea that one has to do something that attempts in a false sense to isolate a particular sub-segment of one's metabolism (because it is popularly assumed that such will benefit one's cardiovascular system) is simply folly, because the cardiovascular system simply doesn't work that way. Indeed, if one takes the time to actually look at the way that the metabolic subsystems of the body function, one will note that if one really wants to maximally stimulate the aerobic pathway one can only do so by maximizing one's anaerobic metabolism. Recall from *Body By Science* that because the glyolytic process (whereby the body converts glucose to pyruvate) can actually cycle much faster than the aerobic process in the mitochondria can accomodate it, pyruvate gets stacked up and gets converted to lactic acid. Consequently, performing anaerobic exercise is the only way in which you can be certain that you have maximally stimulated the aerobic system and caused it to cycle as fast as it can possibly cycle. And in terms of performing a more steady state cycling of the Krebs Cycle at a slower speed, one must remember that when one stops performing one's anaerobic exercise the lactic acid that has been produced through the anaerobic activity now must be converted back into pyruvate. And it is during this conversion process that it is metabolized through the aerobic cycle in a slow, steady state fashion. In other words, you don't have to jog along a busy street, or plod along on a treadmill for an hour to involve your aerobic system – this same steady-state aerobic metabolism takes place when you have concluded your anaerobic workout and are now in a process of recovery. With high-intensity strength training, then, one can be engaging in something productive (such as spending time with your family, working and earning more money or studying for a PhD), while one's metabolic pathways are paying back the oxygen debt that one's muscles have incurred via the anaerobic activity. In other words, the perceived "health" benefit that so many believe only the performance of steady-state activity can provide, actually occurs in the recovery period after high-intensity training with the difference being that only high-intensity training (unlike its lower intensity, steady state counterparts) can actually address your musculature, and, as a consequence, serve to maximize its functional capability. And this has much more of a direct bearing on all of the body's health parameters. It bears repeating that the only way that one can access all of the subsystems of the body (including the aerobic system) is by performing mechanical work with muscles and strength training is a much more efficient and more productive means of addressing the mechanical function of muscles (and all of the metabolic pathways that serve them) than any other (lesser) modality of exercise.

STRENGTH TRAINING – A CARDIO PROTECTIVE MODE OF EXERCISE

QUESTION: I understand your explanation of strength training from the self-evident perspective of human physiology and biochemistry, but what about the scientific literature? Have we, in fact, any proof of these positive cardiovascular effects from studies that have been properly conducted?

ANSWER: The answer is (as one might expect given that the facts of physiology are just that: *facts*) yes. In one very significant study subjects had a catheter inserted into the central circulation so that cardiovascular changes could be measured directly. [3] The subjects tested were stable patients and patients with congestive heart failure. Measurements were taken while they performed resistance training on a leg press machine. Both groups showed beneficial changes in cardiac parameters, but this was more pronounced in the stable group of patients. More important than the differences between the groups was the actual effect on the cardiovascular system: There were significant increases in heart rate, diastolic pulmonary artery pressure (a measure of venous return and end diastolic pressure and thus, indirectly a measure of coronary blood flow), as well as an increase in cardiac index (which is cardiac output per unit of body surface area). Even at the highest workloads, they found a *decrease* in systemic vascular resistance, which resulted in an increased cardiac index and enhanced left ventricular function. In other words, all of the explanations for why V02max might fall off during resistance training did *not* occur. Indeed, what the researchers found out was that the cardiovascular parameters were the exact opposite of what most "experts" had been warning against. It had been believed contracting muscle is going to be squeezing on the peripheral arteries, which would cause increased peripheral vascular resistance, which, in turn, would cause the heart to have to pump against more resistance, thus driving blood pressure sky high and produce a dangerous strain on the heart. And if one really understands the physiology of the cardiovascular system one will realize that this is a completely backwards assumption. During high-intensity exercise there is an outpouring of catecholamines, such as adrenaline (Epinephrine or Norepinephrine) and these hormones act upon the heart and the blood vessels. However, there are different receptors out on the periphery of the body that respond to these hormones in a different fashion. During high-intensity exercise, these hormones act on the blood vessels in the splancnic circulation of the intestines and liver to cause *vasoconstriction*, meaning that the blood vessels constrict and blood flow to those areas decreases. But receptors on blood vessels in working muscles, such as in the pulmonary tree in the lungs, do exactly the opposite: they *vasodilate*, thus allowing for more blood flow in order to supply the working musculature. The net effect being that there's more vasodilation than there is vasoconstriction and, therefore, peripheral vascular resistance, as a whole, is actually lower. And this means that the heart actually is required to pump against *less* resistance, not *more*. When this fact is coupled with the fact that the intensely contracting musculature serves to milk venous blood back towards the heart, and that doing so increases the amount of blood that's delivered to the right side of the heart, which directly determines the amount of blood that is ejected from the left side of the heart, one can see that cardiac output is actually augmented by the increased venous return from the intense muscular contractions. And since blood is ejected from the left ventricle when the heart contracts, when the heart relaxes, that same amount of blood washes in a backwards direction towards the aorta with a closed aortic valve. At the base of the aortic valve are little holes that open into the coronary arteries that supply the heart muscle with blood. Consequently, to the extent that one has an increased venous return, there is as a direct consequence an increase in the amount of blood that is ejected from the left side of the heart, and this increases the amount of blood that back flows into the coronary arteries. So high-intensity strength training not only decreases peripheral vascular resistance because of the dilated blood vessels in the working musculature, but is also augments venous return, which therefore augments end diastolic pressure on the left side of the heart, which augments coronary artery blood flow, which allows for a higher level of exertion to occur with an enhanced blood flow through the coronary arteries. This phenomenon, exclusive as it is to high-intensity muscular work, underscores why proper strength training is the safest form of exercise to perform for people at cardiovascular risk. However, there are more studies to consider in support of this:

A study that was conducted in 1996 provided some interesting data as many experts have appealed to studies to show that resistance training causes unfavorable changes in cardiovascular parameters and lipid profiles. This perpetuated the myth that "weight training is bad for your heart". Studies that supported this notion never tried to factor the contribution that steroid use may have had to the data. This study sought to control for this factor. It seems that the steroid users were the ones with the negative cardiac effects and they were skewing the data. The conclusion of the experimenters was that, "Resistance training in the absence of steroid use results in the same positive effects on cardiac dimensions, diastolic function, and blood lipids as aerobic training." [4]

STRENGTH TRAINING SAFER THAN TREADMILLS

An article that was published in the *Journal of Cardiopulmonary Rehabilitation* examined circuit weight training at varying levels of intensity in patients with CAD. They actually noted a lower rate-pressure product when compared to treadmill walking and no subject displayed any ST-segment depression or angina during circuit weight training.[5] This actually parallels my own experience training patients with known CAD. Despite training these subjects at very high-intensity, taking every set to muscular failure, we have never had a subject experience angina. This is even true for subjects who have angina climbing steps or walking uphill. I believe that the augmented venous return improves coronary perfusion and permits a more meaningful level of exertion in these patients. Resistance training has even been shown to be safe early after myocardial infarction (again, I believe for similar reasons). An article from the March-April *Journal of Cardiopulmonary Rehabilitation* looked at resistance training as early as 6 weeks post MI and compared it to more traditional aerobic-based rehab protocols. Amazingly, they noted that, "30 of 42 subjects had one or more cardiovascular complication (arrhythmia, angina, ischemia, hypertension, hypotension) during the aerobic exercises as compared to only 1 subject with complications during resistive exercises." [6]

-- Doug McGuff, MD

We're seeing now that all of the beneficial changes that can be produced by traditional cardiovascular exercise (and which were previously thought not to occur with resistance training) are actually produced to an even greater degree with high-intensity resistance training. Furthermore, all of the potential dangers to the cardiovascular system such as increased blood pressure and heart strain that have been attributed to resistance training have actually turned out to be nothing more than myth. For people with coronary artery disease, resistance training may prove to be the safest and most effective way to improve their cardiovascular health. As it turns out this is not just our opinion. There are numerous research studies that show that resistance training is safe for those with coronary artery disease and even safe for those who have recently had heart attacks. The cardiovascular improvements that have been obtained with resistance training have been equal or better than those seen with traditional (i.e., low-intensity, steady state) cardiac rehabilitation modalities. In a position paper published in Sports Medicine, the authors concluded:

Circuit weight training has been recommended and has been reported to improve strength, lean body mass, self-efficacy, and may decrease risk factors for coronary artery disease. There appears to be considerable benefit and minimal risk of resistive exercise training for patients with cardiovascular impairment. This mode of exercise may allow patients to perform daily strength tasks safely, more efficiently, and with greater self-confidence. [7]

In another study that examined the effects of a high-intensity strength training program on patients that were enrolled in an outpatient cardiac rehabilitation program, the experiments divided the subjects into two groups, contrasted randomly, with one group assigned to a high-intensity training protocol and the other group assigned a flexibility training protocol. It was noted by the experimenters that the high-intensity training group lost more body fat, gained lean tissue, and improved their treadmill time. Improvements in flexibility were the same in both groups, and the high-intensity training group experienced no cardiac ischemia or arrhythmia during their training sessions. Thus, the high-intensity training group produced all of the improvements with none of the risks. [8] Yet another study of the effects of weight training on women aged 60 to 77, revealed that on a follow up treadmill test conducted with and without a weight load of 40 percent of their bodyweight, the women who took part in the 16-week strength training program showed a reduced heart rate, lower systolic blood pressure, and a lower rate pressure product. The experimenters concluded that strength training reduced cardiovascular stress during daily tasks in healthy older women. [9]

ENLARGED HEART AND WEIGHT TRAINING

QUESTION: Isn't it true that weight training can enlarge your heart?

ANSWER: Although not as common a lament presently as in years past, the refrain that "weight training will enlarge your heart" still endures in some circles (and even among some physicians). The condition this refers to is called ischemic hypertrophic subaortic stenosis (IHSS). This occurs when an enlarged ventricle does not allow blood to flow out of the aorta and fatal heart dysrhythmias can occur. This condition can be seen in athletes, particularly strength athletes. It is the authors' suspicion that the condition is probably related to steroid abuse in those with a congenital abnormality. Along these lines, a study that addressed the question of whether long term resistance training caused heart enlargement was conducted. Echocardiograms were performed on 21 elite male powerlifters and 10 control subjects with the result that none of the powerlifters showed any sign of heart enlargement. Powerlifters do not perform resistance exercise in the manner we have advocated, instead attempting maximum lifts of the heaviest weight they can lift (a modality of exercise that would be more conducive to causing heart enlargement). Despite this fact the researcher in this study concluded that, "contrary to common beliefs, long term resistance training as performed by elite male power-lifters does not alter LV morphology." [10] Study after study has been conducted, all of which reveal in unambiguous terms that resistance training is safe and beneficial not only for enhancing cardiovascular fitness levels, but also a preferred modality of training for those with cardiac disease. [11, 12, 13, 14, 15, 16, 17, 18]

THE SIGNIFICANCE OF VENOUS RETURN

QUESTION: You keep mentioning the issue of "Venous Return" as being important. Why?

ANSWER: The most important thing to realize with regard to cardiovascular protection is that the issue of enhanced venous return is hugely significant, as the degree to which one can enhance venous return is the degree to which one enhances coronary artery blood flow. This is why people with known coronary disease are safer performing proper strength training than they are performing treadmill based aerobic training. While it may be true that conventional aerobic training is less intense, it still raises the oxygen demand for the muscles and the oxygen demand for the myocardium. However, with low-intensity muscular work the muscular contractions are not particularly intense and thus do not augment the venous return nearly as much as properly performed high-intensity strength training does. As a consequence, low-intensity "cardio" exercise increases oxygen demand, but the amount of venous return coming back to the heart is not as great, and, therefore, the augmentation of coronary artery blood flow is not as great. This can create a situation where there can be a mismatch between oxygen demand and oxygen delivery via the coronary arteries – and that's how one can develop coronary ischemia, chest pain, and cardiac arrhythmias – conditions that are *very* dangerous.

THE "BIG 5" AND CORONARY REHAB

QUESTION: Would the "Big 5" program you advocate in Body By Science be a good one for a post coronary patient to follow?

ANSWER: A properly supervised high-intensity strength training program is permissive for a meaningful level of exertion in the post cardiac patient for reasons that we have discussed and that we have illustrated in *Body By Science*. Indeed, the type of rehab that we advocate enhances venous return, enhances coronary artery blood flow and produces a type of conditioning that's actually cardio protective. We are presently witnessing a shift in the paradigm in rehabilitation from a low-intensity, steady state (purely aerobic) rehab program and the notion that strength training is bad and dangerous, to one that is now embracing both with a new emphasis on strength training. However, the pendulum is continuing to swing in the direction where the conventional aerobic component will continue to be de-emphasized (and possibly even eventually dropped) in favor of a more appropriate strength-training program. The "Big 5" strength training program that we advocate in *Body By Science* is both productive and (for the post coronary patient) safe. As far as precautions go for the post coronary patient, we would advise any training be performed in conjunction with the patient's cardiologist. The post coronary patient needs to have a post event stress test that has indicated that he is capable of exerting himself safely, irrespective of whether he's had an angioplasty, is being managed medically, or has had coronary surgery. It is imperative that the patient has a period of recovery, and that he be released by his or her physician to perform exercise. In concert with a physician's approval, we would advise that the client work with a knowledgeable trainer who will work the post coronary patient up to a point of positive failure on each exercise (and we would advise that the patient help in defining this boundary). While exertion that attends high-intensity training is (by its very nature) always uncomfortable and unpleasant, what the patient should seek to avoid (and what the trainer should keep tabs on) is any undue shortness of breath, any chest pain or chest pressure, nausea, and skin that feels unduly clammy or diaphoretic – all of these are markers of potential coronary ischemia. The patient should keep his antenna up for these symptoms. If any of these occur, then the workout needs to be aborted and more medical evaluation needs to occur (this is what happens in any other rehab program and what would need to happen if one is training a patient that was post-coronary event). In other words, one must be sensitive to coronary symptoms, both specific and obvious, and general and subtle. It's best to error on the side of caution in such matters, but shy of these symptoms the post-coronary patient should train in the same manner as anyone else.

HIGH CHOLESTEROL/BLOOD PRESSURE PROBLEMS

QUESTION: I have high blood pressure and high cholesterol problems. Should I consult with my physician before starting the Body By Science *program – and will it help me to control these conditions over time?*

ANSWER: Yes, people who are suffering from high cholesterol or high blood pressure should seek their physician's approval prior to starting an exercise program. For reasons discussed in *Body By Science* regarding metabolism and the metabolic syndrome, issues such as high cholesterol and high blood pressure can often be reversed by a course of proper strength training in conjunction with an appropriate diet that is based on natural foodstuffs. Conditions such as elevated triglyceride levels can be actually be reversed simply by improving one's insulin sensitivity. If someone is a non-insulin dependent diabetic or is on blood sugar medicine, he or she may find that these conditions may well improve as a result of being on a proper strength training program. This is both good and bad; good, in the sense that their condition is improving to a point where he or she may not require as much (or any) medication; and bad in that all of a sudden the former prescribed dosage of insulin that used to barely manage one's blood sugar may now be making one become hypoglycemic. This is another reason why both the patient and the patient's physician need to be aware that the patient's requirement for medication for such chronic conditions may have to be decreased; i.e., the patient may need less blood pressure medicine, he may be able to go off his cholesterol medicine, he may need less blood sugar medicine (or go off of it). Consequently, the patient will need to be monitoring these levels as he proceeds with his training. Indeed, the patient's condition may improve to the point where these medications can actually produce a negative side effect. In terms of the effect of strength training on high blood pressure levels, the scientific literature is replete with data supporting strength training's positive effects. And while we have commonly heard warnings from medical experts that weight training may cause elevation of blood pressure and, thus, should be avoided by people with high (or borderline high) blood pressure, this would appear to be a caveat that is without scientific support. A six-month study that was conducted on 21 borderline hypertensive subjects over the age of 65 proved to be most enlightening in this regard. The subjects performed whole-body weight training involving 7 exercises. At the end of the six months, all of the subjects showed improvement in their blood pressure. To quote the researchers' conclusion:

> The changes in resting BP noted in the present study represent a shift from the high normal category to the normal category. [19]

In the year 2000 a meta-analysis was performed that looked at the effects of progressive resistance exercise and resting blood pressure. A meta-analysis is an attempt to look at *every* quality study that addresses a particular subject. The pooling of data that occurs in a meta-analysis provides greater numbers of study subjects, which, in turn, gives more power to the study's conclusions. With thousands of study subjects, the probability that the study's results where due to chance alone become much smaller. The criteria to make it into this particular meta-analysis included:

- Trials that included a randomized non-exercising control group.
- Progressive resistance exercise as the only intervention.
- Adult humans.
- Journal articles, dissertations, and Masters papers published in English-language literature.
- Studies published between January 1996 and December 1998.
- Resting systolic and/or diastolic blood pressure assessed.
- Training studies lasting a minimum of 4 weeks.

These criteria assured that only the best objective studies were included. The conclusion of this meta-analysis was that "progressive resistance exercise is efficacious for reducing resting systolic and diastolic blood pressure in adults." [20] Even though the above studies indicated that resistance training improves blood pressure in people with borderline hypertension, they didn't really address the concern as to whether or not blood pressure could rise to dangerous levels *during* the workout itself. The answer to this came as a result of a 9-week resistance training study that was conducted that involved 10 experimental and 16 control subjects. At the conclusion of the study marked increases in strength were noted, but, more importantly, the researcher's concluded that, "circuit weight training does not exacerbate resting or *exercise* blood pressure." [21] Despite the evidence presented in the above studies revealing that resistance training actually improves blood pressure, many have argued that these are not necessarily meaningful studies because the studies themselves were only weeks or months long. Such critics have suggested that it is long term weight training as performed by athletes or bodybuilders that is the cause of the blood pressure problems. However, these critics were proven to be in error after the results of a study in which blood pressure was measured both at rest and during exercise between two groups – one was made up of *long-term* bodybuilders, the other being an age-matched control group. The researchers concluded that, "intense long-term strength training, as performed by bodybuilders, does not constitute a potential cardiovascular risk factor." [22] We know now that even during the throes of high-intensity muscular exertion blood pressure is not as high as once feared. Indeed, during a study that examined 16 middle aged men with a history of myocardial infarction, coronary bypass, ventricular arrhythmias, angioplasty and other cardiac conditions who engaged in circuit strength training, it was discovered that the blood pressure data revealed no change in mean systolic or diastolic blood pressure during actual training. This caused the experimenters to conclude that, "In no instance did circuit training appear to elevate a patient's blood pressure above clinically acceptable levels for controlled hypertension." [23] Additional studies have revealed that high-intensity training [24, 25] and even high-intensity muscular exertion, [26] are safe and effective remedies for those suffering from high blood pressure. And while physiotherapists are helpful in rehabilitating many of the conditions we have indicated, many of their treatments could be made much more effective if they employed proper high-intensity strength training. This only makes sense, as no patient is served by being weaker and proper resistance exercise will not only strengthen the muscles, tendons and metabolic pathways but can do so more efficiently and thoroughly than any alternative therapeutic modality.

In October of 1996, while playing in a senior softball game, I was injured in a collision at second base. The surgery to repair the damage involved replacing part of the head of the tibia with a bone graft from my hip and inserting screws in the shaft of the split tibia. In the spring of 1997 I began therapy on my leg. At first I went to a sports medicine facility. However, I was not satisfied with my progress and decided to try rehab at home. This entailed about an hour a day seven days a week. While I felt I was making some progress it was very time consuming. When I learned of the *Body By Science* program, after consulting with my surgeon, I signed up at Dr. McGuff's facility in April of 1998. This proved to be so successful that I have stayed with the program for the last ten years. The injury was so severe that I am still required to wear a brace full time. However, due in no small part to my following the exercise program at Ultimate Exercise, I am able to lead a very active life. I volunteer two days a week at the Emergency Room of the local hospital, play golf once a week, hike, kayak, and do most of the other things a 73 year old would like to be able to do.

-- Charles Sconce (client, Ultimate Exercise, Seneca, SC)

SENIORS AND AQUABICS

QUESTION: My mother is in her 70s and was recently diagnosed with severe osteoporosis. I've told her about Body By Science and the value of strength training to improving her condition, but she was told by a fitness professional at the local YMCA that she would be better served with an aquabics program. What are your thoughts?

ANSWER: Water aerobics for the elderly is the ultimate extension of the argument of fragility of the elderly people, and ends up producing a completely worthless form of exercise. When NASA sends astronauts into outer space, they find that they lose bone mineral density. Similarly, when you submerge yourself into another weightless environment, it does not "load" the muscles and the bones to which they attach in any meaningful way. The percentage of time doing that is not meaningful enough to perhaps diminish bone mineral density (as seniors typically only do it for an hour or so three times a week), but it is a waste of time and it also reinforces the belief in the person's mind that they are "fragile" and that this is the only thing that they are suitable for doing. Doug once saw a physical therapist's note in a chart saying, "Not suitable for land-based exercise." And to us that means that this person belongs in a casket. So aquabics is the ultimate extension of a bad premise, and it's much worse for seniors than having them train too lightly and go through the motions with weights. Aquabics is essentially going through the motions with absolutely no load on the muscles whatsoever – the very opposite of what is required to attempt to remedy osteoporosis. Moreover, most of the people that you see engaging in Aquabics are so fat that they are very buoyant, with the result that there really is no weight bearing taking place whatsoever.

VARICOSE VEINS

QUESTION: Does Body By Science cover any information concerning using your training methods to help varicose veins? I like to strength train and most on-line information about exercise for varicose veins begins and ends with walking. Is the slower cadence strength-training that you recommend in Body By Science okay for varicose veins? I've had them for years and I don't have any pain from them. They just look unsightly.

ANSWER: Not specifically, but the slow cadence we advocate in *Body By Science* really "milks" the deep veins which decompresses varicose veins to some extent. Not a cure, but an improvement.

KNEE REPLACMENT REHAB

QUESTION: I have a client at my gym that has had knee replacement surgery (in fact, he's had two of them). And, of course, the physiotherapists are big on handing out photocopied sheets advocating various stretches that the patient is supposed to do "to get stronger and more range" into various bodyparts. As a consequence of this advice this guy now wants to get on a Nautilus leg extension and put enough weight on the movement arm so that it forces his leg back beyond ninety degrees. I think that's a potentially dangerous thing, but the client believes if he doesn't do it he loses range in his knee joint. Am I right about this?

ANSWER: Absolutely. It's our opinion that some physical

therapists want their patients to do those things (particularly early in the post operative period) to prevent the development of synichae (scar tissue connective bands that can bind the knee up). And this is a procedure that should be done during this period but done manually and gently -- not with a piece of resistance equipment. Particularly not with a Leg Extension machine, because, as we mentioned earlier, most Leg Extension machines provide movement around a single axis point, like the axle of a car. If you look at the femur and the tibia you will note that there is a curved surface that the tibia moves on, so that the rotation of the knee is brought about via a sliding track rather than a single axis. That is to say that it that moves in a curvilinear fashion. So when you activate the knee joint while on a Leg Extension machine that has a single axis, and you flex greater than 90-degrees, that single axis does not match the sliding axis at the knee joint and a crow bar effect takes place within the knee joint. This lever effect can actually separate and damage the knee joint. The individual you mention would be better served by not going beyond 90-degrees and just focusing on strengthening the muscles that surround the knee joint. Think of a diseased joint as you would a rusty hinge on a door; nothing is going to change the fact that the hinge is rusty, and you can do all the stretching of that hinge that you want, but it's still a rusty hinge joint. And that joint can be moved by either weak muscles or strong muscles, and the stronger the muscles that move it, the greater the capability of moving that rusty hinge through its full range of motion will be. And what we find helpful in rehabilitating knee replacements is to first put the client on the Leg Press machine with "0" resistance. Then we'll ask him or her to demonstrate to us a comfortable range of motion for them to operate in. Once this is established we will then pin the machine out so that the client is loaded only through that comfortable range of motion. And after we work them out for a few weeks, we will then expand his or her range of motion by one pin hole in both directions. After a couple more weeks we will then expand the client's range by one more pin hole, and, within eight to ten weeks, he or she will now be using a very meaningful resistance through a full range of motion and have maximal flexibility. It should be pointed out that flexibility is more defined by a functional strength of the surrounding supporting musculature than it is by the pathology (or lack of it) in any particular joint.

PART FOUR: TRAINING ISSUES

SHAKEY LIMBS

QUESTION: *When I approach positive failure on my exercises I note that my limbs begin to shake (sometimes really dramatically). Why does this happen -- and is it a dangerous thing?*

ANSWER: Ken Hutchins (creator of the SuperSlow protocol) was the first person to answer this question. When an individual's muscles start shaking or twitching during an intense set of exercise it is a result of (if we may borrow from mechanical engineering) pulse modulation. The reason for this shaking is that when one is recruiting motor units to perform work not all of those motor units engage at once. For instance, when one is recruiting slow-twitch motor units, one doesn't recruit all of one's slow-twitch motor units simultaneously; one recruits them in a rapid, alternating fashion. Let's say you have 10,000 motor units in a given muscle, comprised of slow, intermediate and fast-twitch fibers. When you begin a set of an exercise, you are typically engaging slow-twitch fibers exclusively, but you're not recruiting all of the slow-twitch motor units at once simultaneously. Some of the motor units are "on" or engaged, and others are "off" or not engaged – and this occurs in a rapidly alternating fashion. This can be compared to the eight pistons of a car engine firing – they're firing rapidly enough so that what would otherwise be a very rough firing of each individual piston is being damped out to produce smooth movement. And the same thing happens with motor units; they fire very rapidly in an alternating fashion like the pistons in the engine of a car. But as you fatigue these motor units and they drop out, you have fewer units that are firing randomly. So it's like a car engine that you start pulling spark plugs out of; if you pull two spark plugs out of an eight-cylinder engine it will then be firing on only six cylinders and the engine will start to run roughly, shaking and jerking. If this process of pulling spark plugs two at a time continues, by the time you have pulled out four more, the engine will only be running on two spark plugs or two cylinders, with the result that the engine will now be running so rough that it will feel like it's going to shake right out of the vehicle. The same situation occurs as you approach muscular failure in an exercise; i.e., your muscles are attempting to produce force (in order to continue lifting a weight) and motor units are dropping out. Consequently, the smoothness that was experienced when you were able to randomly fire 10,000 motor units has by the time you get to your last two repetitions been diminished to the random firing of only 50 motor units. And the random firing of 50 motor units is too low a number of motor units to damp out that roughness, with the result that your limbs (like the engine) begin to shake, which is the biological equivalent of the pulse modulation of that engine when it's running roughly. And just like the shaking of the eight cylinder car engine that is reduced to running on two cylinders, the random firing of those motor units in your muscle actually starts to become visible. This phenomenon becomes particularly evident if you're using a piece of equipment that has a long movement arm, such as a Compound Row or Chest Press machine, as the vibration from one's shaking limbs becomes amplified through the long flexible movement arm of the machine, making the tremors that much more apparent. However, this is an absolutely normal by-product of muscular fatigue and nothing to worry about. In fact, it's a good indication that you are working out with the level of effort necessary to ensure that you are doing everything that you can to stimulate a positive adaptive response. It's nothing to be avoided or worried about.

SORENESS

QUESTION: *I am a personal trainer in a crowded workout center. Often times after a workout that is performed along the lines that you have advocated I'll have a client that says that he "didn't really feel anything" after his workout. The attitude seems to be that if he doesn't feel sore the next day, he didn't have a good workout. What are your thoughts on the relevance of soreness to a productive, growth-stimulating workout?*

ANSWER: Soreness definitely doesn't have any direct correlation to growth stimulation. It's simply a potential by-product of having performed a workout that was meaningful. Sometimes you will have significant soreness after a workout and other times you won't. It should be pointed out that if you are sore after a workout, this doesn't mean that growth has taken place once the soreness goes away. It simply means that you're no longer sore; not that you've recovered from your previous workout nor that you're ready to train again (i.e., that you've fully recovered and overcompensated from your previous workout). Most times you will find soreness occurring in movements that involve the muscle contracting over or around a boney prominence. For instance, it's not uncommon for a trainee to experience soreness the day after a workout in which Squats or Leg Presses had been performed. In such instances, the trainee will experience soreness in the buttock muscles as a result of the fact that during these exercises not only are the buttock muscles heavily involved, but also because the buttocks are contracting while actively being pulled taut over the protuberance of the ischial tuberosity. A similar phenomenon will be noted after performing a pulldown exercise, which a lot of times will cause soreness in the latissimus dorsi muscles not simply because of the work that the latissimus performed in the movement, but because the tip of the scapula digs into the belly of the latisimus muscle while one is performing the movement, in such a way that the muscle is actually contracting over a boney prominence. It's not unlike taking a steak and stretching it over the edge of a granite countertop. In other words, the soreness that is produced after a workout doesn't necessarily have a correlation with anything. We know of many women, for instance, that love doing barbell lunges because they think it works their buttocks so well. But really all they're doing is taking their ischium bone and jamming it into their gluteus muscle and causing mechanical damage. The truth is that soreness is not a valid measure of anything but soreness. You could make your quadriceps sore simply by working them over with a ball-peen hammer, but that, likewise, wouldn't necessarily correlate with anything productive having been stimulated. Your client needs to get rid of the notion of soreness being meaningful. We understand that a degree of soreness can make you feel like you've been worked and that something has happened and, consequently, can be a positive post-workout experience for a lot of people – but please don't take it to be the *sine qua non* of a workout's effectiveness because there is really no data to correlate that notion at all. The only way you can determine if you've made progress (shy of a body composition measurement) is whether or not your workout chart indicates that you are stronger.

STASIS IS RETROGRESSION

QUESTION: I'm a high-intensity personal trainer and was very intrigued by your statement that if you attempt to "hold" a client at a given weight and Time Under Load that he will regress. I have a couple of clients that have indicated that they're happy with their present level of size and strength and wish to stay at that – what should I do?

ANSWER: Attempt to continue to progress them. Whenever we have attempted to hold a client at a given weight and Time Under Load he has or she has invariably retrogressed. It appears that the body is able to calculate that the challenge it is facing is not escalating, so the adaptation that been produced as a result of progression, now starts to deconstruct. In this respect the body is like a bicycle; i.e., you cannot balance on a bicycle unless you're moving. And unless you're moving forward the body's adaptive machinery it does not work well, as its response mechanism is finely tuned to new and increasing challenges. So, from our vantage point, it's very important to continue to progress your clients, even if you're just progressing them up by a quarter of a pound on a particular exercise.

INVERSE COMPLIANCE PROBLEMS

QUESTION: I have a client that is making amazing progress with the Body By Science program. I think that he will make even better progress by spreading out his recovery days between workouts to 10 (from 7). The thing is that he wants to go in the other direction – he wants me to train him two or three times a week in the belief that he will double or triple his progress! What do you think I should do?

ANSWER: We would suggest that you – at least – hold him to once a week and keep a close eye on his progress chart. If his progress stops, then it may be time to reduce his workouts to a "Big 3" or a Split Routine along the lines advocated in Chapter Seven of *Body By Science*. Your question brings up a problem that we have observed with certain of our own clients over the years. Namely, what skews the data and affects all of the popular books and fitness magazines that are currently in vogue is what we refer to as an Inverse Compliance Problem. To digress for a moment, when considering prescription techniques for most medications, if the physician simplifies the dosing regimen and decreases the dosing regimen, compliance goes up. If you have a pill that has to be taken three times a day (such as an antibiotic that has to be taken three or four times a day), as opposed to a once-a-day antibiotic, the compliance for the once a day antibiotic is always better than with the multi-dosing regimen. For instance, if you have a birth control pill that has to be taken 21 out of 28 days as opposed to a birth control patch that you wear for three weeks at a time, you'll find that the compliance rate with the patch is much better than with something you have to remember every day. So, generally, compliance improves as the dosing frequency *decreases*, but in the realm of physical conditioning we've found that the better responders will suffer a drop off in compliance if their frequency is not at a certain level. And we believe this is the case because the good responders get such positive feedback from the training experience that they misidentify the stimulus-organism-response relationship. In other words, they have come to think of exercise as directly *producing* the result they display because that result came so quickly and dramatically for them. Nevertheless, in our opinion, the dosing interval is still more advantageous for most clients when it is spaced further apart, despite the fact that many better responding clients clamor to workout more frequently. As a trainer, you're between a rock and a hard place as if you stick to you guns (which you should) and don't capitulate to their demand they will simply do it elsewhere and/or quit coming to your facility. And in terms of data, such individuals simply blow the curve for frequency because they just can't restrain themselves. It's very rare to find a good responder that does not want to train more frequently. However, most good responders are not the ones seeking out all that science has to offer to get the most out of their training as they believe (based on their results) that they simply don't need such information. The vast majority that do not possess such genetics most certainly do need such information and the good news for them is that when no one else or no other popular training approach could coax results out of their bodies, the *Body By Science* approach can. And it can do this because it takes into account just how long it takes people to recover and produce an adaptation. And for the poorer responders it can be a long time. Indeed, some of our poorest responders require a minimum of 12 days to elapse between workouts before they show improvement, and training them any more frequently than this results in retrogression. And this is particularly true for people that are average or poor responders and that also have stressful lifestyles – i.e., rotating shift work, small children requiring attention and/or something that produces a significant stress and/or disruption of sleep cycles. Such trainees simply must train with less volume and frequency in order to produce results because human adaptive energy is not just dedicated to one's workout; it's dedicated to one's entire life. Someone that is embroiled in a lawsuit, or going through a divorce, or taking care of an ill parent, all of these things will delay that person's recovery ability as each life event makes significant demands upon one's limited reserves of adaptive energy.

THE "BEST" WAY TO TRAIN

QUESTION: I loved reading Body By Science! *The training and fat loss information made perfect sense and I'm getting leaner and stronger with each workout. I know that you advocate different protocols as one gets more advanced, but is the "Big 5" workout taken to positive failure the best way to exercise? I think so!*

ANSWER: While we advocate a protocol of strength training that has a scientifically validated track record of success, we want to guard against being prescriptive of any *one* particular strength training protocol as being "best," simply because there are multiple different factors of the stimulus we seek, and as one progresses and improves, different components of the stimulus may become more or less important to one's growth and development. Sometimes in order to get more of one component of the stimulus, one will have to sacrifice another component, so one may need to cycle back and forth between different protocols to get the maximal benefit out of every different component of the stimulus. For instance, to the degree that you're going to emphasize the component of *accumulated by-products of fatigue* (such as lactic acid), you may have to sacrifice the load component to some degree. Say, for instance, you're using a slow contraction protocol and going for a longer Time Under Load; to some degree you're going to have to sacrifice the component of load in order to accumulate a lot of by-products of fatigue. Conversely, if you want to emphasize the *load* component of the stimulus you may wish to employ the Max Contraction protocol whereby the muscles are trained in their fully-contracted position for 5-to-15-seconds of exertion. This will have you sacrificing a percentage of the accumulated by-products of fatigue component in order to achieve this. And if you're going to go all the way up to Omega Set or Negative-Only training, then the metabolic by-products of fatigue component may be sacrificed still further in order to employ even greater loads. Our approach, then, is to make the workout demanding physiologically, but within an environment in which certain issues such as force are controlled and the trainee is able to go to a point of legitimate muscular failure. This, so to speak, is represents the hub of the wheel. Attached to that hub are many different spokes, each representing different components of the total stimulus. However, every time we emphasize a different spoke of the stimulus -- whatever it may be – it has been our experience that doing so always takes a disproportionate toll on one's recovery. And even if you are going to use a slow lifting technique that produces a deep inroad, you have to be aware that a very little bit of such training is going to necessitate a large reduction in both the volume and frequency of such training in order for it to prove beneficial. You have to realize when you're adjusting your protocol you're kind of playing with dynamite and you have to dose it appropriately. It is important to remember that the stimulus is comprised of many factors that cannot be infinitely reduced down to a solitary component. And all of these segments make up the totality of the stimulus, and no one of them contains all of them.

LOOKING AT "LOAD"

QUESTION: I'm interested in getting bigger, so should I just focus on the load or micro-trauma component of the stimulus?

ANSWER: Not exclusively. We do know that micro-trauma to the tissues is a by-product of the stimulus that contributes to the growth process, but it doesn't follow that one should just aim to create micro-damage – for instance, engaging in Negative-Only work will cause damage to the cross-bridges within muscle tissue, but a steady diet of Negative-Only exercise will put you too much onto the catabolic side of the equation and create an overtraining situation very quickly that will take you months to recover from. Remember that the stimulus must always be considered within a specific context that balances the catabolic with the anabolic, and this context is multi-factorial and complex. Moreover, it must be remembered that not every cause produces a proportionate effect; that is, some causes can produce a gigantic effect on recovery ability, whereas other causes produce a much smaller effect, but an additive effect to some degree. If it's muscle growth you're after then load will certainly be a huge component of the stimulus you're seeking, but load is also one of the components we indicated that produces a BIG effect on one's recovery ability. And with an increase in muscle mass as your primary goal, don't forget that other components of the stimulus factor into the "mass" equation as additive components that, while perhaps not as significant as the load component in building mass or hypertrophy, nevertheless contribute to muscle growth as part of the overall context. So, if you look at all of the modes of progression that we have outlined in *Body By Science* you will note that all aspects of the stimulus should be tapped for optimal growth and development.

MULTIPLE SETS

QUESTION: What is wrong with performing multiple sets during training (where you perform several sets per bodypart and several exercises per bodypart)?

ANSWER: People that perform multiple sets per muscle group simply misunderstand what the stimulus is for the response that they're seeking. Once one has recruited all of the motor units that one is capable of recruiting and has fatigued them out, one has really done all that one can do in terms of imposing the necessary stimulus. The problem is that in order to perform a high volume of muscular work (such as multiple set) one has to actually hold back on the amount of intensity that one is investing into that muscular work in order to achieve a high volume of it. So what happens is that one never reaches the level of stimulus/intensity required to trigger the adaptive response that one is seeking, but instead accumulates an amount of work that will chronically interfere with -- and quite possibly prevent -- the adaptive response they seek from occurring.

PERIODIZATION

QUESTION: What are your thoughts on the training concept of periodization (where you train intensely for some periods of the year and less intensely and more frequently during other times of the year)?

ANSWER: "Periodization" is an attempt to over-complicate what is a relatively simple process. The concept of "Periodization" seems to be have advanced for no other reason than to make the people who have advanced it appear to be intelligent. When one states that there are different training approaches (all apparently involving 3 sets of various repetitions) that are responsible for building "mass," "strength" and "strength and size" (and, in one training certification course, another method for building "hypertrophy" as against "size"), one is simply wrong from a physiological perspective, and simply suggesting scenarios that simply have no bearing on how the body actually works. These are just silly categories of activity that are being assigned and that are just arbitrary in their titles. Certain advocates of periodization claim that by training less intensely one is engaged in what they call "active rest," which is an oxymoron, particularly when what is really required is simply "rest." If one has applied the proper stimulus, then one's body needs to be left undisturbed long enough for it to produce an adaptive response, which is difficult at the best of times. Again, if you go back to the grocery store and you look at that pound of ground beef and consider the fact that your body has to produce that amount of tissue almost out of thin air, you are better able to realize that in order for your body to accomplish this it will need to be undisturbed for a period of time just to be able to do it. But if you keep throwing in workouts of varying degrees of intensity (the so-called "active rest" periods) you're really just interfering with your body's ability to produce such an adaptive response.

A BROAD SPECTRUM OF RECOVERY ABILITY

QUESTION: Why do you think there is such a broad range of exercise tolerance and recovery ability among individuals -- particularly given the universality of our species' musculoskeletal system?

ANSWER: When you ask that question you actually have to look at the nature of evolutionary biology in general, as opposed to looking at it from an "Intelligent Design" standpoint. If one makes the cognitive error of thinking, "Well this *should* be an intelligent design, so why don't we all respond the same way?" – then, not surprisingly, one will end up confused and frustrated with their training. Evolutionary biology, however, operates from a different viewpoint; i.e., that our bodily responses are not the result of design but rather purely accidental. A single base substitution on a DNA molecule can completely change the expression of a gene altogether. And those single base substitutions can occur randomly and as a result of exposure to environmental elements, and this results in an organism that is *basically* the same but has a broad expression of different physical characteristics and capabilities. Over time, for both the organism and for the species as a whole, this produces adaptive advantages that allow for the propagation of that particular species. And from a biological standpoint, this variation in our metabolic capabilities yields a tremendous benefit for a species. In our species' history, for example, we hunted and gathered in tribes or bands of 25 to 50 people. Consequently, it was to the band's decided advantage to have two or three people in the band who were extraordinarily gifted in endurance activities, and to have one or two people who were extraordinarily gifted in strength activities. Such diversity contributed enormously to the survival of the entire band, as if there were two people who were really gifted in endurance activity they could be used to chase down an animal until it became exhausted and could be killed for food. After it was killed it had to be dragged or carried back to the campsite for everyone in the band to share, and, consequently it was to the band's decided advantage to have two members who were metabolically adapted to be very strong. So having a huge spectrum of metabolic versatility, particularly in an animal that evolved as a hunter-gatherer, is an extraordinary adaptive advantage for a species. And from an evolutionary biology standpoint, this is also why we possess this wide range of adaptability in our species. However, most people in our species fall in the middle of a bell curve in terms of their response patterns to the exercise stimulus, but many that are within the middle of this curve desire the characteristics of the extremely strong individuals that are 2 Standard Deviations to the right of this curve. They want to try to emulate these outliers and to produce results that will make them more like them when it's simply not in their genetic cards to look like that or to share these characteristics to the same degree. But in terms of why that wide variation of metabolic capabilities exists across a particular species, the simple answer is that such variation produces an adaptation that benefits our species as a whole.

"EXPLOSIVE" TRAINING

QUESTION: *I'm an athlete and I need explosive power when I'm competing – particularly in changing direction quickly. Don't I need to train explosively in order to develop this power? I mean it would seem that training slow will make me slow, whereas training fast and explosively will make me fast and explosive. What are your thoughts on this?*

ANSWER: This is a common question posed by most athletes that require power in their game – from hockey to football. Remember that it is your fastest twitch motor units that are able to produce explosiveness and speed. So by the capability of tapping into your fastest twitch motor units and making them stronger and larger, you will increase your ability to be *explosive* and fast. This refers to the concept of *capability*. And explosiveness, in our opinion, is made up of two things – *capability* and *intent*. Intent is a neurological event; an electrical impulse traveling from your brain to the motor unit in question. And intent is comprised of two things: one is the genetic component of neurological efficiency and quickness and the other is rehearsal and practice. And both the rehearsal and practice need to be very specific to the sport or activity you will need this explosiveness for. For instance, BMX racers are very explosive; they can get out of a starting gate with incredible explosiveness, quickness and amazing twitch velocity, but if you had them try to express that in getting off the line in a 40-yard dash, you wouldn't be particularly impressed. The reason being that the skill set that they have rehearsed and practiced in order for them to be explosive is *specific* to that skill set alone. So if there is an activity that one wants to be particularly fast, explosive and quick at, one needs rehearsal and practice of that particular activity. But one also needs *capability,* and capability is produced by strengthening the fast-twitch motor units that are going to be called into play during the sport or activity in question. But to say that getting at those fast-twitch motor units by slow, controlled repetitions that result in sequential motor unit recruitment is going to make you slow is a supposition contrary to fact. The people who make such assertions, as far as we can ascertain, have no real data to support their contention. They're engaging in circular reasoning because what they use to measure "explosiveness" is the very same skill that they practice in their training. If, for instance, one is trained in an "explosive" or ballistic fashion with weights, and then tested by EMG, one would do well in the test because one would have rehearsed that particular skill. And if one trains in a manner that we advocate in order to strengthen one's fast-twitch motor units and then is allowed to rehearse the movement that will be used in the testing of explosiveness, you will find that one will have become more explosive in expressing one's power. But make no mistake, it is not training quickly or explosively that results in explosiveness being developed in a particular skill, but rather the rehearsal of the specific explosive activity that one wants to use as the measuring stick. And what's happened in the studies that these people cite is that explosive training was also the measurement tool that they used to measure the subjects' "explosiveness." If someone trains in a way that results in sequential recruitment and strengthening of the fast-twitch motor units, and then is allowed to rehearse the means of measurement specifically –they will, in our experience, express superior results. One of the authors (Doug McGuff) is friends with Mike Bradley, who is the strength coach of Florida State University's basketball team. Bradlely trains his players in a high-intensity fashion and they have no problem with sprint speed, explosive changes in direction or their vertical jump. To improve their explosiveness in the vertical jump, for instance, the players simply perform their high-intensity strength training and practice basketball. And these results are produced by a training program that doesn't risk injury, which is an important consideration for athletes as there are more athletes injured as a result of their training programs than there are injured as a result of competing in their sport.

"STABILIZER" MUSCLES

QUESTION: *What you have suggested makes a lot of sense. However, I note that you don't suggest any free weight exercises. How, then, does one develop the stabilizer muscles?*

ANSWER: The deep muscles surrounding your spine and your internal abdominal cavity are typically referred to as "stabilizers." But having acknowledged this, one must also acknowledge that any muscle can be a stabilizer. To serve as a stabilizer a muscle simply has to be contracting statically. If, for instance, one is leaning against a wall, one is using one's quadriceps as stabilizer muscles by contracting them isometrically as one holds oneself up. As the way to improve a muscle in both of its functions –dynamic and static – is to produce an exercise stimulus that involves moving that muscle through a reasonable range of motion and inducing a rate of fatigue that results in a stimulus for growth. This can be applied to any set of muscles, including muscles that people commonly think of as "stabilizer muscles," such as the lumbar muscles and the abdominal muscles. But to suggest that they need to be approached differently because they possess a stabilizing function simply isn't accurate and, consequently, is not necessary. The abdominals are addressed more than adequately with the "Big 5" routine. When muscles start to fatigue in an exercise such as Pulldowns, the muscles that are in that kinetic chain, including the abdominal muscles, will be very heavily involved, making it unnecessary to perform any supplemental exercises in order to obtain maximal development from them. The whole concept of "stabilizer muscles" has been popularized mostly as a marketing ploy for different training concepts and different types of training equipment. And the whole concept of "core training" is a marketing mechanism for selling devices to train the abdominal muscles, which everyone seems to be fixated on. Most people are fixated on them because they have either a conscious or subconscious belief in the "spot reduction" theory (i.e., that if you can lose bodyfat from a given area by exercising it directly). All that aside, every muscle in the body – from the flexor of your pinky finger, to your rectus abdominus muscle, to your trapezius muscle – i.e., any muscle that you can name can be a "stabilizer muscle." And the way that we think of it is that a muscle is either contracting isotonically, meaning its contracting under load and shortening; it can contract eccentrically, meaning it is contracting under load and lengthening, or it can contract isometrically, in which case the muscle is actively contracting but not producing movement. Any muscle that is contracting isometrically, therefore, is acting as a stabilizer. The whole concept of "stabilizers" or bringing stabilizers into play while you're actively working another muscle is just a romantic notion that really doesn't have a reference in reality. There isn't a class of muscle known as "stabilizer" muscles. Any muscle can be a "stabilizer" if it's contracting isometrically to stabilize the body from any opposing movement in the opposite direction.

TRAINING BY "FEEL"

QUESTION: Many trainees advocate training by "feel" (i.e., how a given muscle feels during an exercise), and if you don't feel it working then you shouldn't do that exercise. They argue that this is a better stimulus than counting reps, Time Under Load (and even the weight used) in a given exercise or exercises. What do you think about this approach – does it have merit?

ANSWER: Given the various genetic determinants of response to exercise, it could well be that those who believe in developing a "feel" for training are of a genotype that speaks that language. If you ever visit the various Internet message boards that discuss exercise you will note that there are those trainees that have found through trial and error something that seems to work quite well for them. For reasons they can't quite articulate their approach typically involves a higher volume than we would advocate and involves the "feel" associated with pumping up their musculature. In our opinion, such people are of a particular genotype mix that responds to such a protocol and thus appeals to them. Unfortunately, like many others in the world of training, once they've found something that has a limited application to those of the same geneotype, they believe that it will apply across the board to *all* geneoptyes and that people who don't agree with them on this (or that fail to produce similar results), "just aren't doing it right" or "just don't understand." It's always good to ask what the denominator is in such instances. For instance, several years back a magazine publisher wrote a book and held a contest that offered thousands of dollars and a brand new Corvette to the person who produced the best results on his training program. Such a prize allowed the publisher to cast out a very wide net and pull in a lot of people with it, which dramatically increased his chance of being able to land a few geneotypes that would respond impressively to his training protocol (of course he then plastered up their pictures as poster children of his "great" training program). But the question you have to ask yourself is how many people bought his book and did his program – but produced "zero" results? The publisher only posted the success stories – not the failures (which were legion). That's the denominator. And how many people were involved in the actual case study – 7, 8, 9? And how many of those people were already bodybuilders (i.e., were those of a genotype that responded easily to any training stimulus and perhaps were consuming anabolic steroids and/or other growth drugs) and were just looking for a venue to obtain exposure for themselves on the Internet or in a book? So, as with all protocols that emphasize one aspect of a multi-factorial process, a thorough training approach does not attempt to reduce the stimulus to one dimension. And if you do resort to a single protocol for a while, some component of what your body will produce is going to be a specific metabolic and skill set adaptation to that particular protocol. In other words, some of the improvement that you're going to see is just going to be you getting better at that particular skill set in the same way that the "aerobic" conditioning that occurs from the skill set of running will completely NOT translate to the skill set of cycling. To some extent, your protocol becomes not just a means to an end, but an end in itself in terms of the specific adaptation to that protocol.

CONSTANT CHANGING OF WORKOUTS

QUESTION: Since the stimulus is multi factorial, wouldn't it be best to change your protocol every single workout?

ANSWER: Not really. We don't subscribe to the notion that some trainee's have embraced; namely, that workouts are like snowflakes; i.e., each one should be different. The reason being that when something's brand new you haven't really been able to make the necessary adjustments to make sure that the intensity of that exercise or protocol has been maximized. When you use new equipment, for instance, you can't really be certain of your weight selection. And then you have to allow a period of time for those adaptations to tap themselves out. It is only once all of the skill set adaptations have been tapped out that, by default, your body will then produce an increase in muscle mass. And this simply requires time to elapse in using a given protocol in order for you to get everything you can get out of a particular protocol. In other words, there has to be some sort of baseline to change from in order for there to be change at all. If change is the constant standard, then that becomes essentially the new routine; the new standard, non-changing event.

THE MULTI FACTORIAL STIMULUS

QUESTION: So what exactly are the various factors or components of the exercise stimulus that need to be accounted for?

ANSWER: Muscle growth is a multi-factorial process that is an offshoot from muscular contraction against a specific load. These factors flow from load – just the muscle being loaded with a significant amount of weight -- in the following ways:

Damage -- The stimulus can sometimes (and in hunter/gatherer times often did) cause minor injury, which brings about positive adaptation through repair, such as when mechanical damage occurs to a muscle through micro-tears in its sarcolemma. This allows for certain growth and repair elements and enzymes to enter the muscle, and thus contribute to the production of a slightly bigger and stronger muscle.

Glycogen Depletion -- Similarly, and perhaps of greater importance for the adaptive process, is the degree of glycogen depletion from the muscle. In studies conducted on distance runners, for example, it has been noted that when their fuel tanks (glycogen stores within a muscle) are drained, their bodies overcompensate by first replenishing the exhausted fuel supply, and then overcompensating by putting back a little bit more than was there initially as a reserve or hedge against future needs and dearths. As water bonds with glycogen at 3 grams of water per 1 gram of glycogen, and since glycogen is stored in the muscle, this explains why muscle is 76 percent water and why glycogen storage plays such a large role in determining the size and energy potential of muscle tissue.

Inroad -- Another key component of the stimulus is inroad; i.e., the momentary weakening of muscles. Inroad is a signature that you are recruiting motor units and fatiguing them in a sequential pattern. When you start off lifting a weight the first motor units you recruit are the smallest motor units and these are composed of slow twitch fibers. As these fatigue and fall out of the equation you'll then move on to recruit intermediate twitch fibers, which are slightly larger motor units. As these fatigue and fall out you will then recruit the largest, fastest twitch motor units and fatigue those out. As that happens, you grow progressively weaker. If you're lifting a weight of 200 pounds, you're strength level starting out may be at 320 pounds. But as you lift and lower that 200 pounds over the course of a set you're recruiting and fatiguing motor units and becoming progressively weaker. When your force output drops to 199 pounds you will have reached muscular failure.

Accumulated By Products of Fatigue -- The metabolic byproducts that accrue as a result of exerting yourself during the inroading process described above are also part of the stimulus. These would include the production of lactic acid and the lowering of pH levels, as these by-products create an environment where certain enzymes and hormones that are part of the growth stimulus come into play.

All of the above factors contribute to the potency of the stimulus and, thus, the long-term effectiveness of one's training program.

GLYCOGEN

QUESTION: I'm intrigued by the role of glycogen depletion as part of the stimulus. Can you elaborate on this?

ANSWER: Certainly. Think of it this way: If one has 100 percent fuel stored in a muscle but one never uses this to capacity, instead using, say, 60 percent consistently in one's workouts or activity levels, then the body will not perceive this is a sufficient stimulus to warrant an enlarging of the energy reserves in that muscle. Indeed, such would be a stimulus to cause the body to conclude that it is wasting a considerable amount of energy simply preserving a bigger "gas tank" than is required, much like a home owner will come to a similar conclusion about the necessity of spending money each month to heat rooms in a large house that are no longer being used. Consequently, such would be a stimulus to *downsize* the existing gas tank by 40 percent of its present capacity, thus causing the previous 60 percent level to now become the organism's 100 percent capacity. It should be pointed out that the body is very frugal when it comes to its energy systems and thus will not waste energy in preserving a tissue size that it does not perceive the necessity of. Instead, it will seek to downsize or conserve energy at every turn. This, in part, explains the sarcopenia (loss of muscle associated with aging) that we witness in our culture. And as muscle size diminishes through the above process, metabolic rates correspondingly decrease and typically do so in an environment in which energy consumption typically stays the same or increases, thus resulting in more calories in and fewer calories out, and the surplus calories being converted to fat, which is then stored in greater and greater quantity on our bodies.

LOAD AS COMMON DENOMINATOR IN EXERCISE

QUESTION: It would appear that Load is the common denominator that has to be present for any type of benefit to be stimulated from exercise. Wouldn't you agree?

ANSWER: It's true that load is the common denominator, particularly in the fiber recruitment process. It was demonstrated clinically in 1973[1] that, at light loads, slow-twitch fibers contract and are capable of sustaining repeated contractions at this relatively low intensity. Since these fibers are weaker, they're not suited to a higher intensity of effort or overload. If a greater load is imposed upon the muscle, a progressive recruitment of larger and stronger (fast-twitch) muscle fibers occurs. Thus, when the load increases from light to heavy there is a progressive increase in the number of muscle fibers involved in the contraction. As we've seen, this may only be relevant within a certain percentage. It can be emphasized to a greater or lesser extent, but without load you really don't have exercise. Even the by-products of fatigue are usually a by-product of lactic acid or pyruvate, and that is really an anaerobic metabolic process that is produced within a specific time frame, which in turn is limited by load. Damage to some degree is a factor, and likewise related to the amount of load your muscles are subjected to as they contract and the same would apply to Inroad as a stimulus borne by contracting against a specific load and then, as a natural course of things, causing the muscle to weaken. So it seems that load is the common denominator as without it, we're not sure that the other factors would exist or be produced from an exercise standpoint. Now having said this, there exists a threshold for load, whereby the rate of fatigue must be such that it results in a sequential (and maximal) recruitment of all of the available muscle fibers and, as a consequence, accumulation of by-products of fatigue. This doesn't necessarily mean that more and more load – regardless of the context – is better, but there is a critical threshold for load in order for this type of exercise to be occurring. And this also doesn't mean that as part of tweaking the stimulus you can't engage in protocols that maximize load. But generally, there has to be a certain minimal amount of load, otherwise you can't generate enough intensity to produce the beneficial effects that we're looking for from exercise.

LOAD AND FIBER RECRUITMENT

QUESTION: What would an optimal load for exercise be?

ANSWER: This will depend largely upon the individual's existing strength levels. Regardless, by the time you are 85 or 90 percent of the way to muscular failure in terms of your Time Under Load, you have probably recruited all the motor units that you're capable of recruiting, and between that 90 and 100 percent, you're probably just optimizing your firing rate of all the recruited motor units that you can until the point where your strength is no longer adequate to move the weight. Indeed, research conducted by S. Grillner and M. Udo [2] indicated that while parallel increases in load and muscle fiber recruitment occur, this process happens only up to a certain threshold point. They observed this threshold to be at 50 percent of a muscle's maximum voluntary contractile ability. In fact, their research indicates that 90 percent of all available muscle fibers in a targeted muscle group have been activated with a load that is roughly 50 percent of a muscle's one-rep maximum. Also, there is evidence that gains in strength obtained from a program utilizing weights in the range of 90 to 100 percent of a subject's one-rep maximum for low (1-

6) repetitions are not necessarily the result of a still greater degree of fiber recruitment. Instead, the strength gains may result from alterations in the pattern of nerve discharge. The research we cited above by H.S. Milner-Brown and colleagues [3] strongly corroborates this notion and goes on to reveal that the discharge of impulses appears to synchronize in response to muscular contraction against resistance close to 100 percent of a muscle's maximum voluntary contractile ability. Evidently what happens in this respect is that the synchronization parlays into better timing between the nerves innervating the muscle and the rate of contraction. This results in the impulses for muscular contraction occurring more or less simultaneously, which heightens the electrical input into the muscle at one time and significantly amplifies the contractile force capacity of the existing fibers, irrespective of their actual size. So, the load you use in your exercises should fall somewhere between 50 and 80 percent of your One-Rep Maximum as a general guideline.

FIBER TYPING AND GENETICS

QUESTION: *Are the genetic traits you have indicated in Chapter Eight of* Body By Science *associated with muscle fiber types or are they something independent of fiber typing? There are, let us say, three major classifications of muscle fibers – slow, intermediate, and fast – are there certain genetic factors linked to these different fiber types, or are they a more or less random occurrence?*

ANSWER: It would appear that they are linked, perhaps not in a direct causal sense, but it has been established that there is definitely a strong association between certain genetic markers and the twitch-velocity of muscle fibers. For instance, the angiotensin converting enzyme (the "ii" version of it) definitely has a strong correlation to slow-twitch fibers as it has more of an endurance profile. Myosin light chain kinase is actually part of the coupling of the contractile proteins, and therefore is expressed in higher concentrations in fast-twitch fibers than it is in slow-twitch fibers. In addition, if one requires more speed or power, one will require more cross bridging and more power output in the fast-twitch fibers, with the result that alpha-actinin-3 is found only in fast-twitch skeletal muscle. So all of these things do correlate very strongly with fiber type and fiber type mix.

CLIENT INPUT AND TRAINING MODALITY

QUESTION: *So the Client should train according to what he or she prefers?*

ANSWER: Not necessarily. We always get a little leery when the term "prefers" comes into it the equation because then that allows the subject's psychology to dictate to a large extent what they "want" to do, and that is always going to fall on the side of lower intensity and lower effort for reasons that we've covered in *Body By Science*. Nevertheless, given our species' natural tendency to conserve energy, we've found that if a person is being supervised appropriately during his workouts he will expend the requisite energy to have a productive workout. In fact, we've found that almost 80 percent of the benefit that comes from having an instructor oversee one's workout comes merely from his presence during the workout. In the presence of a knowledgeable instructor, people that would otherwise prefer to avoid exertion will make the extra effort necessary to inroad properly. Nevertheless, while a trainee shouldn't necessarily train according to how he or she "prefers," both the trainee and the trainer should pay close attention to their progress chart. As if a trainee starts to display better results from working with a slightly lighter weight or a longer Time Under Load (or something that is a little less intense but allows for a little more volume), then we would advise both trainee and trainer not to ignore this, because that may be the direction necessary to produce the trainee's best response from high-intensity exercise.

THE NAUTILUS INROAD MODEL AND GENETICS

QUESTION: *Would it behoove a trainee to use the old Nautilus formula for determining optimal repetition ranges? Arthur Jones believed that a 20 percent inroad into one's starting level of strength was sufficient to stimulate optimal increases in one's size and strength. What are your thoughts on this?*

ANSWER: We believe that Arthur was basing his conclusion on his own personal experience –which we all tend to do. But if, for instance, we choose a resistance for someone to work out with that is 80 percent of their 1-Rep-Max, and this subject has a low expression of Myosin light chain kinase, he might be able to create a 12 or 15 percent inroad into his starting level of strength. But a second subject who has very high levels of Myosin light chain kinase who works out with that same 80 percent of his 1-Rep-Max, might discover that, upon failure, he has created an 85 percent inroad into his starting level of strength. So genetics can really muddy the water on such simplistic inroad formulas. Moreover, if you took someone with high expressions of Myosin Light Chain Kinase and tried to make up a protocol wherein he was only going to inroad 20 or 25 percent, you may find that he would have to use such a ridiculously light weight that he would never reach positive failure, and, thus, never receive a meaningful stimulus from his exercise sessions. So our short answer to that is that the old Nautilus formula may not have as broad an applicability as we once thought. Now having said this, it might provide some degree of insight into what type of genetic endowment a person possesses, or at least suggest a direction that such a person might want to consider taking with his training. But, in general, we've found that if one shoots for a mean, issues such as the ideal depth of inroad will start to declare themselves. And they start to declare themselves based on how much inroading seems evident when they're training. One of the simplest things to do to determine if someone is a big inroader or a small inroader is to go to failure at one's given weight (which typically falls in that 80 percent of 1-Rep-Max range), and then immediately cut the weight by half. If one is a moderate inroader, one should be able to continue with the exercise for another 30 seconds (Time Under Load) before one fails again. If one doesn't inroad very deeply at all – which may be an expression of one's level of Myosin Light Chain Kinase – one may continue on for a minute and a half or two minutes before reaching failure. But if someone is a really deep inroader you can take him to failure, then drop the weight 50 percent and have him try again and he may go 10 or 15-seconds -- and he'll be done. What we've found is that in terms of subjects, their performance and their preference almost self-select for the best inroading protocol.

THE "NOT-TO-FAILURE" WORKOUT CONCEPT

QUESTION: I've read recently about inserting a "Not-To-Failure" workout into one's weekly routine, whereby you don't go to muscular failure but this allows one to keep one's training frequency up. This evidently provides an "active rest" to the muscles, which keeps them stimulated but not overtrained. What are your thoughts on this concept?

ANSWER: We addressed the issue of "Active Recovery" elsewhere in this chapter. However, we believe that the human muscular system requires a stimulus of a specific nature and magnitude in order to warrant an adaptive response by the body. In the context of muscle building, the nature and magnitude of the stimulus is 100 percent of a muscle's (or a group of muscles') momentary ability, culminating in a state of muscular failure. By definition, other stimuli that do not meet the criteria do not pack the same adaptive stimulus. Once we have determined this to be the best stimulus, we know from evolutionary biology that this is a necessary force driving the adaptive mechanism and that has to occur (or be applied) relatively infrequently to allow for full recovery of the higher order fibers. We further know that the frequency of such exposure has to be such that these higher order fibers have sufficient opportunity to recover and adapt. The idea of a "not-to-failure" workout seems to us a justification for the unfounded belief that one must workout more than once a week. And the only justification for this belief seems to be tradition based (i.e., "that's the way the most massively muscled bodybuilding champions trained before steroids came on the scene"), rather than evidence based. It also fails to take into account the fact that the "champions" were (and are) the genetic freaks (in terms of recovery ability and ability to grow muscle) of their respective eras. We certainly don't see a need to train two to three times a week. Further, such claims about what allegedly happened in the "old school" of bodybuilding; i.e., how bodybuilders typically trained in the 1930s, 1940s and 1950s, is simply not supported by the historical evidence. If you have access to any of the yellow pamphlets that were put out by Peary Rader, or the 20-Rep Squat program, you will note that these are very consolidated routines that were recommended to be performed once a week (or less in a lot of cases), as this was the formula that the authorities of the day found effective for the general population. A lot of the three times per week thinking came out of Nautilus during the Arthur Jones era, as Arthur found that two to three weekly workouts produced results in not only Arthur, but also in many of the superb athletes that went to DeLand, Florida to train under his supervision (such as professional football players and competitive bodybuilders). However, Nautilus itself was a black swan in terms of how it appealed to the collegiate and professional athletic community, which, along with the time and place in which it flourished, created a selection bias for drawing the type of people to their headquarters that could tolerate higher volumes of exercise. However, from a review of the literature "active rest" is not a spoke on the stimulus wheel and, thus, is not a requirement for stimulating muscle growth. And after a workout the trainee's body needs to recover his resources, which it can only do during "rest" not during "activity."

THE MUSCULO-METABOLIC MISMATCH

QUESTION: Do you see any context in which not training to failure might be helpful to the growth process?

ANSWER: The only context in which we would envision such an event as perhaps being helpful would be in situations where an individual has pushed his training out to the point where he is working out but once every two to four weeks. Under such a scenario, it is possible for the lower order fibers to decondition somewhat during this time frame, and, thus, a workout that is not intense enough to recruit the faster twitch motor units might allow those fibers the additional recovery time they need while paying service to the shorter recovery requirements of the lower order motor units. For instance, we have noted that as a trainee consolidates his routine in order to continue to progress in strength there arises an inability by the trainee to tolerate the requisite dosing. In other words, if we took a very advanced subject who was performing two or three sets perhaps once every 12 to 14 days, they would still continue to grow stronger, but then get to a point where they were terminating their workout for metabolic reasons. This is a phenomenon that we have dubbed a "musculo-metabolic mismatch," owing to the fact that the muscular strength component (i.e., the structural component) occurs over a different and more protracted time frame than do metabolic adjustments.

What made this hit home to me was when I read a case report in the Emergency Medical literature of a man from Machu Piccu who came to visit Los Angeles because he was thinking of moving there. He spent his entire life living at very high altitude, came to Los Angeles for two weeks, went back home afterwards -- and died of high altitude cerebral edema because all the metabolic components of adapting to altitude went away completely during that two week time span. And it dawned on me that the Slow and Intermediate Twitch motor units have enzymatic capabilities that have to be conditioned and ramped up in order to carry you to the point where you can *then* activate

Fast Twitch motor units. And as you get stronger, all three motor unit types improve their respective functional capabilities, but the Fast Twitch motor units are going to improve to a greater degree. Thus, the amount of anaerobic punishment and the accumulated by-products of fatigue that you must bring to the organism will grow greater as you get stronger, which, in turn, requires longer periods of recovery. However if the dosing interval is stepped out to 10 days to two weeks, you will now be at a dosing interval that may cause the metabolic adaptations of the Slow and Intermediate Twitch motor units (the ones that carry you up to that level of tapping the Fast Twitch fibers) to deteriorate. And, as a trainer, you want to continue to progress your clients in their training, and so you must escalate the stimulus dose and begin to space out their workouts to bring to them an escalating dose but less frequently to allow for full recovery. However, the dosing interval may now be spaced out so far that the metabolic adaptations that had taken place within the Slow and Intermediate Twitch fibers (the effective bridge in a sequential recruitment to the Fast Twitch fibers) at a once a week frequency, now begin to decondition, and the "bridge" is no longer there. And you will find at this point that the client will become nauseous and short of breath, as a result of having lost that component of metabolic adaptation necessary to carry them to the full recruitment of the Fast Twitch motor units.

-- Doug McGuff, MD

So, as one begins pushing their workouts out two and three weeks apart from each other, one might require a protocol to be interspersed at 7-day intervals of a stimulus/intensity that is of a level sufficient to maintain the metabolic adaptations of the Slow and Intermediate Twitch motor units, but not intense enough to fully tap the Fast Twitch motor units. The structural components of the Fast Twitch motor units are maintained for many weeks, but the metabolic adaptations that take place in the lower order muscle fibers are not structural elements, but synthesized chemicals that can ramp up and ramp down very quickly. And when a trainee's workouts get to the point where the stimulus is applied so infrequently, the metabolic adaptations ramp down quickly, and the accumulated by-products of fatigue component of the stimulus can now cross the narrow therapeutic window and become a toxic component that inhibits one from tapping the full potential of the stimulus. It may be that nobody needs to perform *any* type of exercise more than once a week, but you may not need to push yourself to the level where you're recruiting and stimulating the Fast Twitch motor units more frequently than once every two to three weeks, as long as once every seven days you are doing something that will preserve the lower order motor units metabolically.

DR. McGUFF ON
THE NAUTILUS NORTH STUDY

QUESTION: I've read John Little's report of his Nautilus North Study and am really impressed by it. However, I was wondering what Dr. McGuff's view of the study was and whether it passed scientific/medical muster?

ANSWER: When we were writing *Body By Science* John asked me the same question, as he was concerned that it wasn't published in a peer-reviewed journal (which was the only reason we did not include it in our book, by the way). And I told him that while it might not have been printed in a peer reviewed journal and that it did not meet all of those criteria, in terms of its methods and how well it was done I thought it was better than just about anything I've seen in the formal literature. And I think the only thing where it lacks sophistication is in statistical analysis, but I think that is decidedly to its advantage because in most of the studies that I've reviewed the experimenters simply take raw data and convert it into a relative percentage change rather than a raw percentage change. And the only way that data can really be meaningful to anyone is if it provides raw numbers. And what John had in his study was raw numbers -- and that's what really matters. For instance, when you read that hormone replacement therapy increased the risk of breast cancer by 25%, everyone freaks out. But when you look at the raw numbers, you note that the increase in risk of breast cancer ranges from 1 in 125,000 to 1 in 100,000, so it's still an infinitesimally small risk in exchange for other benefits that are occurring that may be of a much larger magnitude. But large numbers of people in the medical world became upset because they were reviewing the relative values that the study reported, not the absolute numbers. So first of all I think the Nautilus North study was very well done; it was performed by knowledgeable people who used very strict criteria -- as opposed to being managed by a graduate student that was reading a magazine while the training was being conducted (as is often the case with studies). And secondly, it reported raw data, which is very important. So I thought that it was an incredible study that really pointed out a training frequency that's optimal for the vast majority of trainees. The only people who are uncomfortable with it are those that don't like the data it contained (as it didn't support their particular prejudices on the matter of training frequency). There has been a huge movement in the bodybuilding and general fitness fields to shout down the people that are trying to argue for a lower frequency, and while we acknowledge that there might be a sub-segment of the population that, because of genetic factors, are better able than most to tolerate a higher frequency of exercise, these are people that a possess a genetic variation whereby they already have a lot of muscle anyways and simply desire to use and display it on a more frequent basis. Ironically, this small percentage of the population have disproportionately influenced the argument in the training frequency debate. But I think the hard data that John presented in the Nautilus North Study was very compelling. And the other thing that came to mind for me when I saw the statistical curves of the data indicating post workout states of below baseline, baseline, and then peaking above baseline (several days later) was why would anyone want to spend more days *below* baseline than *above* baseline? Why would one want to have more days where one is subnormal in functional ability as opposed to having more days when one is supra-normal?

PASSIVE INSUFFICIENCY ISSUES

QUESTION: *I like what you said in* Body By Science *about passive insufficiency in forearm training. Are there any other muscles groups where this plays a role?*

ANSWER: You will note a similar phenomenon occurring if you don't sit properly in a Leg Extension machine. If you're sitting bolt upright with your hips flexed at 90-degrees, you'll discover that you can't fully extend your legs. If you sit up in your chair with your back at 90-degrees right now and try to do a Leg Extension, you'll note that you can't get those last 10-degrees of extension, but if you lean back in your chair just 15-degrees then you can fully lock your knees. That's another example of passive insufficiency occurring because your hamstrings are partially contracted when you're sitting bolt upright and this prevents your quadriceps from fully contracting. Also, there is *Active* insufficiency of the rectus femoris muscle in this position. Because this component of the quadriceps is fully contracted, the other heads of the quads cannot shorten further. Leaning back at the hip also gives the rectus a little more room to shorten so the other heads of the quadriceps can be fully engaged.

REP CADENCE

QUESTION: *I don't have Nautilus or MedX machines. Should I still use a Superslow* ™ *style of protocol for my exercises?*

ANSWER: While we like Superslow ™, the protocol doesn't have to be Superslow ™ to be effective. We think of Superslow ™ as being the spirit of the law, rather than the letter of the law for the simple fact that the equipment that many people are going to have available to them will often preclude the use of such a slow protocol. Given the incorrect strength curves on some pieces of equipment, if you're going to go for 10-seconds up and 10-seconds down (ala Superslow ™), then you will end up shutting down the exercise prematurely simply because of a mismatch between what your muscles are capable of and a need for momentum to get through a particular sticking point. It basically has to boil down to moving as slowly as possible as you can without becoming herky-jerky. On some optimal pieces of equipment that will indeed be a 10-seconds up and 10-seconds down cadence, but even this will depend upon a trainee's neurological efficiency. We have clients where if you try to get them to move any slower than 5-seconds up and 5-seconds down, it just gets too herky-jerky to be productive or efficient. So on some pieces of equipment (and for some subjects) it's going to be 15-seconds up and 15-seconds down, and on less ideal pieces of equipment it may be 4- seconds up and 4-seconds down.

FREE WEIGHTS & CONVENTIONAL EQUIPMENT

QUESTION: Do you have any recommendations for trainees who use mostly free weights in their workouts?

ANSWER: The biggest issues with free weights and other exercise machines are effective loading of the muscles and sticking point issues that are more related to the mechanics of the equipment than muscular fatigue. To some extent sticking points with conventional equipment might upset the cadence you might use, but we would still advise that you contract your muscles as slowly as you can possibly go without your set deteriorating into a series of stops and starts. For instance, in exercises such as the Barbell Squat, in the lower turnaround position (i.e., at the bottom of the movement when your thighs are horizontal to the ground) you will find that the load is way heavier than it is at the top position and, thus, the tendency is going to be to spend time lingering during the easy part and speeding up during the hard part. However, you should really focus on doing the opposite; i.e., you should really attempt to slow down and linger through the difficult part and not lollygag in the easy part. And this should apply to all free weight exercises you might perform. The cadence in such exercises may vary somewhat, depending upon where you are in the range of motion of the exercise, but the emphasis should always be to move as slowly as you can without the movements deteriorating into a series of stops and starts, and should also be performed in such a way so as to make the movement as difficult as possible rather than as easy as possible.

COMPARING NAUTILUS AND MEDX LEG PRESSES

QUESTION: What is the difference between a Nautilus Duo Squat/Leg Press and the MedX Leg Press? I go to a gym that has both, but I don't know if I should use one or the other.

ANSWER: Both are good machines, so you're training options are excellent. The differences are largely in the cam profiles. The Nautilus Duo Leg Press has a negative cam, which makes its stroke significantly different from the MedX Leg Press. The MedX Leg Press, set at a one-foot stroke with 600 pounds results in 600 foot pounds, while most other Leg Presses move through a two-foot stroke, so the same 600 pounds on the weight stack translates into 1,200 foot pounds, so comparisons of Leg Press machines are not an apples-to-apples kind of thing. But, more importantly, on the Nautilus Duo Leg Press/Squat the negative cam unwinds so that when your legs are fully extended the amount of weight that is borne by the hips, lower back and knees is almost infinitely more than it is at the beginning of the movement. By contrast, the MedX Leg Press has a four-bar linkage system with the resulting difference in leverage being that the sticking point in the machine is approximately four-inches out from the start of the movement and then, after that, there is a pretty rapid fall off and the movement becomes easy.

DON'T LEG PRESS UNILATERALLY

QUESTION: On the old Nautilus Duo-Squat and Duo-Leg Press machines, you have the option of training one leg at a time or unilaterally. Is this something that you would recommend or is this too much of an exaggerated range of motion?

ANSWER: We're not particularly big fans of unilateral loading of the legs because it creates some significant loading differentiation and rotation around the pelvis. If one leg is in the portion of the range of motion where it is almost completely locked out, the resulting loading through the pelvis is completely different than it is for the opposite leg that is fully drawn back, with the result that you are getting some rotation around the pelvis that unequally loads the lumbar spine and makes it a little bit prone toward tweaking your back. This is augmented considerably if you are using the Duo-Squat because what happens then is that you have the negative cam come into effect, so in one extremity you have the cam completely unwound, which almost infinitely increases the load on that side of the spine, while on the other side, where the leg is fully flexed, the cam is completely wound. The result is that the resistance on the one side is almost infinitely less than it is on the opposing side, and you now have a really heavy, unequal loading of the spine. We know that many people that have a Nautilus Duo Squat or Duo Leg Press have fused the movement arms together so that the machine can only be used bilaterally and this prevents the unequal loading. We think the Nautilus Duo-Squat and Duo Leg Press machines, in terms of generating intensity and really giving the legs a great workout is excellent, but it also produces unequal loading around the spine with the rotation of the pelvis that occurs and this can put the trainee at some risk for tweaking his back.

TRAINERS AND BILLABLE HOURS

QUESTION: *My personal trainer, who is very well versed in high-intensity training, insists that I workout twice a week. I notice that my progress has slowed down over the past three months. Shouldn't I be training once a week by now?*

ANSWER: If your trainer is from our recommended list of facilities, our inclination is to trust that trainer's professional judgment. We recommend once a week as a good starting point and that frequency should be decreased as a first mechanism to deal with slow-downs in progress. However, your instructor may alter your frequency as a means of uncovering if you are one of the relatively rare subjects who responds better to more volume or frequency. If, however, twice-a-week training seems to be a matter of rote for your facility it may be that financial issues are driving the training frequency more than the data on your workout card. If your progress has been poor for three months ask your instructor (and yourself):

1.) Am I getting stronger?
2.) Are my measurements improving?
3.) Is my body composition improving?
4.) Do I feel good more days than I feel spent?

If the answers to any of these questions is "no", then we would recommend a reduction in training frequency as a measure of first resort. If, after several rounds of reduction in training frequency, results are still not forthcoming, then other alterations in protocol may be required.

MAX CONTRACTION

QUESTION: *I've heard that training with Max Contraction or Static Holds will only develop the muscle and strength in the range in which the contraction is performed – not throughout the whole muscle. I believe that Arthur Jones tested this and found that there was a general (Type G) response and a Specific (Type S) response to static type exercise. If this is true, what would be the upside of building up only one part of the muscle to the detriment of the rest of the muscle?*

ANSWER: This is a specious argument because motor units distribute their fibers homogeneously throughout the length of a muscle. So as you start to recruit high threshold motor units, you're doing so homogeneously throughout the whole distribution of the muscle. As a result, the Type S and the Type G responses that Arthur

Jones talked about are more of a neurological event. Consequently, if you've spent some time training your muscles through a regular range of motion rep and then go to a Max Contraction Training protocol (as we suggest in Chapter 7 of *Body By Science*), then you will produce a strength increase throughout the entire muscle.

TRADITION

QUESTION: *I love your scientific approach to training. My question is why isn't this taught in "Exercise Science" classes at university? I go to a school that has an exercise science class and they are still teaching the position that you have to perform low-intensity steady state activity for "cardio," stretching for flexibility and strength training three days a week. Why don't they teach a real science-based approach to exercise such as what you advocate?*

ANSWER: We suppose that what is popularly taught as exercise science is really, for the most part, folklore inherited from coaching circles and various exercise traditions and beliefs. In this respect, it's not dissimilar to teaching theology. There is a subject matter; there is a body of knowledge that has been laid down and that can be learned and that one can have mastery of -- even though it can be based on a complete non-existence of facts (since faith does not require proof). If you're a theologian you're teaching people about something that is not testable or based on observable evidence, but nevertheless comprises a massive body of knowledge with lots and lots of texts. And we liken the same thing to a lot of what's going on in the universities with exercise physiology classes, among other things that are presently going on in the universities. They do have mastery of a known existent body of knowledge – it just happens to be largely wrong and not adequately supported by basic science. And this includes published physiologists who claim that you have to do your "cardio" separately, and also published "authorities" who are adamant that you cannot get cardio from strength training and that it needs to be performed separately.

And these are gentlemen with PhDs affixed to their names, an indication that they have put in time and have learned the body of knowledge that has been passed down (however inaccurate it may be) to the satisfaction of their professors. And now it is their turn to pass along what they have learned to another generation of misinformed students of their "denomination" of exercise science. When you're raised in the Church it's possible for you to become more secular, but I think it's really hard to make the break, particularly when your bread is still buttered by the Church. Michelangelo did great Renaissance work but he did it all within the context of the Church because that's where he was trapped. And likewise if you're an academician in an exercise physiology department, we don't think that you can be iconoclastic and survive. Consequently, the old traditions are what are taught in the exercise science classes, rather than concepts that run counter to these traditions -- even when the old traditions have been proven false and often harmful.

PULLDOWNS & PECS

QUESTION: In Body By Science you state that one of the muscle groups that is strongly involved in the Pulldown exercise is the pectoral muscles. How can this be?

ANSWER: It's just the way human anatomy operates. If you're a doubter and if you're used to doing your Chest Press exercise early in your workout, try doing a set of Pulldowns as we've described them to muscular failure and then go immediately to your Chest Press. If you've been operating under the assumption that you haven't yet worked your pecs, you'll be surprised to find that your Time Under Load in the Chest Press with a given weight will be significantly down because of the involvement of the pecs on the Pulldown movement.

ABS

QUESTION: Why don't you include any direct abdominal work in your "Big 5" workout?

ANSWER: Because then it would be a "Big 6" workout (just kidding). A lot of people think that they have to do a sit-up or a crunch to really work one's abdominal muscles, but the rectus adominus muscle is a linear muscle that contracts in a linear fashion and only shortens the distance between the lower sternum and the pubis by a short distance – and this is completely incorporated and accounted for by performing the Pulldown (particularly with the slumping motion that we recommend for this exercise).

DEEPER INROADING

QUESTION: In looking at the videos on www.bodybyscience.net I note that you have your clients (and even yourselves) continue to push for a 10-second static hold after they have reached positive failure. This looks demanding! Do you do this each and every workout?

ANSWER: Yes, particularly with beginning clients, we'll have them continue to push for a 10 count. What will happen is, based on our judgment and whether they're able to hold the load statically or if the negative is starting to take them over, that count to 10 may be relatively slow or we may accelerate it depending upon how that client is behaving under load. But we do have them continue to push, not so much because we think there is a heightened stimulus from doing this deep inroad technique, but (particularly with the beginning and intermediate clients) doing so helps us to make certain that the positive failure the client displays is truly a state of positive failure. If we have them perform a deep inroad technique at the end of their set where they're pushing as hard as they can -- and the negative is beginning to overtake them -- we can be fairly certain that the failure they reached was bona fide.

CLIENT ANGST

QUESTION: Do you ever have a client get angry with you because they're sore the next day as a result of *training in the* Body By Science *fashion? After all, it is very demanding!*

ANSWER: Not that we can recall. And you're right that the *Body By Science* workout is demanding, but it is the very demanding nature of it that makes it so productive and so time efficient, so most of our clients consider the occasional soreness they experience as an equitable trade off for the results they gain from the workouts and the time that they save. Moreover, soreness has not been a huge, huge issue with most of our clients. We do tell them that if they experience an undue amount of soreness from a particular workout that they are welcome to come back for a second workout, which, for reasons we don't fully understand, seems to relieve soreness (for whatever reason, producing movement in the same plane that they previously used in their workout seems to obviate their soreness to a significant degree). But for the most part, we don't really note undue soreness as being a significant complaint. This may be because the "Big 5" workout consists of big compound movements, and is performed over an appropriate range of motion for our clients (rather than an *excessive* range of motion). By contrast, if you have someone perform a Leg Press where their knees are crammed up to their ears and they're jamming the boney prominences into their buttocks and overstretching things, or if you have them perform a Chest Press exercise where the stretched position is greatly exaggerated, then, under those circumstances you may have a client experience excessive soreness. You see this happen with large women who go to conventional trainers or aerobics studios, where the instructors will have them perform exercises such as Lunges, the act of which jams the bone in their buttocks into their gluteus maximus muscle and will produce undue soreness. By contrast, the fact that we don't have a degree of soreness that might otherwise be expected is because we are placing people in a biomechanically appropriate movement with an appropriate range of motion so that they do not get the degree of mechanical stretch damage that occurs when they exercise improperly.

HOW MANY EXERCISES?

QUESTION: *I'm a personal trainer and, having supervised hundreds of workouts personally, I've noted that when one of my client's gets beyond a "beginner" level, having them perform more than three exercises in a single workout -- and still have them be able to do justice to each of the exercises they perform -- is impossible. At some point they reach a diminishing returns threshold where they find themselves giving 100 percent to each exercise, but they no longer have 100 percent to give. And if the trigger point to stimulate an adaptive response in a given muscle is, say, 100 pounds for 10 repetitions, when you give them that same 100 pounds on exercise number four, they may only be able to perform five repetitions – which is five repetitions below the trigger point for that muscle group. Do you agree?*

ANSWER: The degree to which this is true is somewhat dependent upon the individual, and the amount of muscle mass that he has at baseline. We believe that there is a critical mass of accumulated by-products of fatigue that can be handled per given unit of time – even with maximal metabolic conditioning. Consequently, if we have a client who is a lean, muscular 220 pounds, we know that he can perform a Leg Pess, a Pulldown and a Chest Press, and if he's really giving it his all and moving briskly from one exercise to the next, you can (in a very well conditioned subject), have a situation where he's spending a half hour on the carpet feeling ill after his workout before you can even get him up off the floor. And that's certainly a possibility. However, if for some reason you wanted to include more volume (which one would have to question why), simply allowing a little bit more time in between exercises will metabolize off some of that lactic acid, and let your client's blood Ph return to a more normal level, with the result that he would be able to better tolerate a little bit more volume than three exercises in his workout (But, again, it's not really clear why you would want to do that anyway). On the flip side, however, is that a smaller subject, say, a female client who weighs 110 pounds, may well be able to perform a fairly significant amount of sets (perhaps five, six or seven in a given workout), before she reaches the point where she's metabolically unable to continue; i.e., where the accumulation of by-products of fatigue and lactic acid is such that when she moves to her final exercise the force of her muscular contractions is now so small as to be insignificant. However, even this lowered force output can be used to a trainee's advantage if you know how. In his *Superslow* ^{TM} *Technical Manual* Ken Hutchins wrote an interesting chapter entitled, *Intensity Versus Work in Exercise*. And the premise of this chapter was to look at a basic five-exercise workout in light of two different scenarios. In Scenario A, each of the exercises is performed with five minutes of rest in between each exercise. In Scenario B, the trainee moves quickly from one exercise to the next with no rest at all in between each exercise. All of the exercises in both scenarios are performed to a point of momentary muscular failure, with the only difference being the rest periods (or lack thereof). Not surprisingly the weights employed during both scenarios were comparable for the first exercise, but with each successive exercise, the trainee who rested longer between sets was able to use more weight in his exercises. However, the accumulated by-products of fatigue component of the stimulus is much greater with Scenario B, resulting in a greater *depth of fatigue* (i.e., inroad). So when you're moving quickly from one exercise to the next, you may experience a drop off in the amount of weight that you can use in your exercises, but that doesn't mean that you're not reaping benefits from doing so. Remember, the stimulus as not an isolated component; it's multi-factorial. The stimulus is a combination of load, accumulated by-products of fatigue and inroad. And the important thing to remember is that over time all three of these elements are important and need to be included in one's training. This is elaborated on in *Body By Science*, revealing how a trainee can alter the protocol to emphasize different aspects of the stimulus over time. As a trainee becomes more advanced, he may benefit more from experiencing greater load at the expense of the inroad and accumulated by-products of fatigue components. Conversely, there will be times during a trainee's career when he will benefit more from the accumulated by-products of fatigue component, which will come at the expense of load and inroad. But when you increase any one of these, you will be sacrificing the other two components to some extent, and the important thing is learning how to intelligently manipulate these various components over time so that you are getting the most stimulus possible but not too much of any one so that you are maximizing your exercise experience.

DOUG McGUFF'S MOST PRODUCTIVE WORKOUT

QUESTION: I have a question for Dr. McGuff. I'm just curious, looking back over all the years that he's been training, what has been Dr. McGuff's most productive workout routine?

ANSWER: My most productive routine (when I was at my biggest and strongest) consisted of three exercises performed once every 12 days. I divided it up into an "A" workout and a "B" workout that consisted of a Leg Press, a Pulldown, and an Overhead Press (Workout "A") and then a Calf Raise, a Deadlift and a Chest Press (Workout "B"). In looking back I note that every time I've made dramatic increases in strength and size, it's always been as a result of reducing the volume and frequency of my workouts. And I have tried upping the volume of my workouts, I've tried the blitz thing – and every time I've done it I've felt like hammered dog crap, I get depressed and I get smaller. In contrast, every time I've reduced the volume and frequency of my workouts I've gotten bigger, healthier and happier.

JOHN LITTLE'S TRAINING

QUESTION: My question is for John Little; you've trained with Mike Mentzer and created several protocols (Power Factor Training, Static Contraction Training and Max Contraction Training). What have you learned about training and recovery over the years and found to be the most effective method for building muscle?

ANSWER: Certainly the most dramatic results I've ever experienced came from using heavy overload partial reps. During the course of one week my bodyweight went up from 178 pounds to 190 pounds – and while this was before I had access to a BodPod, given that I didn't consume anything beyond my normal diet at that point, I am left to believe that the bulk of the gain was muscle weight. The best results I've ever seen were on a client who used Max Contraction, and gained over 6 pounds of muscle in one week (and this time I did have access to a BodPod to test his composition). However, for total fitness and health I like a "Big 3" or "Big 1" workout performed with a pyramiding of static holds, the "Done In One" protocol or a dynamic protocol of "Big 3" exercises using a slow cadence. As a side note, when I took part in the Nautilus North Study I used Mike Mentzer's Infitonic protocol and the resulting data revealed that it was 11 days before any growth was produced. And being someone who likes to train, the prospect of waiting 11 days didn't sit well with me. So I experimented with a version of Mentzer's Ideal Routine wherein I trained chest and back together, took seven days off, trained shoulders and arms, took another seven days off and then trained legs. My reasoning was that by training only a third of the body each workout (as opposed to a whole body workout), my recovery period might be quicker. I did this for three months and during this time measured my results every day in the Bod Pod to see what the data revealed as to when I should train again. And even with this protocol nothing showed up on the Bod Pod until day 10! I then experimented on myself with one set of negative only exercise and was stunned to learn that it still took my body 11 days before anything in the way of a lean tissue gain showed up. So, after several years of extensive compositional testing on myself I've learned that I must take between 10 to 11 days off between my workouts (almost irrespective of what training modality I use). That's simply how long it takes for my body to produce anything in the way of an adaptation. And I found that to be true even with once a week training; i.e., if I try to workout once a week and perform three or four exercises to positive failure, the next week I may use those same exercises and I might be up a rep on one, I'll hold on another and go down on another. In other words, I'm not fully recovering with only seven days off in between my workouts. And this was brought home vividly to me by training my 17-year-old son, who started training at age 16. He'd been training once a week on a split routine and, at age 17, his metabolic machinery is very receptive to the workout stimulus. As I'd been struggling with increasing my reps on the Nautilus Leg Press for months, I changed over to a three way split such as my son was using whereby I trained my legs every third workout and, with three weeks off in between leg workouts, I shot past my previous best repetition record in the leg press by 15 reps per leg! And it dawned on me that there is something hugely important about the recovery side of the equation. And the only thing I can attribute this to is that when you train a muscle group to failure, especially a big muscle group like the legs, it is comparable to draining an Olympic size swimming pool and attempting to fill it back up with a garden hose – in other words, it's going to take a long time. Perhaps 3 weeks. By contrast, training the biceps is like draining a little plastic wading pool that you might get at WalMart; that is, you might be able to refill it in a day. So, while my experience might be considered extensive in some circles, I'm still learning more each year. And the more I learn, the more it impacts my training. I will say that nothing I've learned has led me away from the primary principles of high-intensity training that were taught to me by the late Mike Mentzer: "Exercise to be productive must be intense, brief and infrequently performed."

AMPLIFICATION CASCADES & ADRENALIN

QUESTION: If adrenaline stimulates an amplification cascade, isn't it true that often adrenaline levels can be spiked by psychological means by people who are scared or nervous or anxious? If so, is the demanding muscular work that we engage in when we train somewhat lessened or damped because of various other adrenaline trigger mechanisms that beset us on a weekly basis?

ANSWER: To some extent, adrenaline is always going to produce that effect, but that effect is really only going to be *significantly* pronounced if there's a real stimulus for it to need to be used. Being anxious will make you spill out adrenaline, and you will cleave some glycogen and some fatty acids as a result, but unless you are actually performing the demanding work that is going to consume those energy mediators that are being released, then you're not going to reap much if any benefit. If they are not being consumed by high-intensity exercise, then their levels are going to quickly build up in the bloodstream, and the balance is going to change such that you're going to quickly revert back to storing those elements (the spilled glucose and fatty acids in the bloodstream). If there's not a high-intensity exercise demand to actually consume these resources when they're released into the bloodstream, then they are going to be quickly restored to a homeostatic level and put back where they were taken out before any significant long-term effect can occur. So it's not just the adrenaline that's important; it's the adrenaline released in the proper context whereby the glucose and fatty acids that have been liberated are actually going to be used as metabolic fuel. Were it otherwise, then you could just simply give someone an injection of speed or ingest amphetamines and have a positive benefit. But doing so wouldn't provide you with the necessary health benefits because while you might be stimulating the system, you are in effect simply putting your car in neutral and revving the engine, so to speak.

A PERFECT EXERCISE ENVIRONMENT

QUESTION: What, in your opinion, would be a "perfect" exercise environment?

ANSWER: Perhaps the best place to start would be with a description of what a perfect exercise environment is *not*. And almost universally what it is not is any commercial gym that you walk into nowadays. Most commercial fitness centers mix up all different forms of exercise within eyeshot of each other (and often within the same space). The typical commercial gym places an emphasis on sustaining a communal or nightclub atmosphere, including lots of multi-media paraphernalia (i.e., TVs everywhere, high tech speakers blaring out music that you may or may not like, lots of neon signage, people reading magazines, newspapers or listening to I-pods while on recumbent bikes or treadmills) and other features that serve only to distract. Very little attention is paid to the quality of the equipment, the maintenance of the equipment, nor is there attention paid to the maintenance of the proper workout environment in terms of such simple things as gym temperature. If one drives by any large commercial gymnasium one is immediately struck by the glass façade that allows one to see into the workout area. And if one then chooses to look inside, one will note that the facility is typically packed to capacity and, should you be able to view the facility's weight training area, it will usually be a mixture of free weights and various machines (typically employing cables and pulleys that don't vary the resistance on the weight stack in synch with the strength curves of the muscles they are supposed to train). Look a little bit closer and you will see roughly ninety percent of the weight room's clientele sitting on benches or leaning against something – i.e., not training. Indeed, the environment in terms of how the exercises are performed in most commercial facilities is a strong negative reinforcement to engaging in the kind of workout that we're advocating (particularly during peak hours when the facility is really crowded). If you do attend a commercial gym, you will find that it is best to do so only during the gym's non-peak hours, so that you can at least get some of the crowd issues out of the way.

BOUTIQUE FITNESS CENTERS

QUESTION: Why do so many people go to such fitness centers?

ANSWER: The reason that most of the clientele have for coming to such fitness centers is no different than the reason that most of them go to Church or that they recycle; i.e., they believe that doing so makes them a better or more complete person. Some also do it to have their ticket punched; that is to say, to meet what they believe are their requirements for looking after the "physical" part of their lives. And this is reflected in a lot of the rules in commercial gyms where they have a "no grunting" policy; that is, if anyone lets out a grunt, groan or a scream during their exercises they are ejected from the facility. And while we're all for stoicism in training, we do have some clients that cannot output maximal effort without some audible indication that effort is involved. And to think that we should punish or eject someone from the facility for exerting the kind of effort that might result in their making progress seems to us simply ridiculous. It's a boutique approach to something that requires effort -- and lots of it. For these reasons, we are not big advocates of going to crowded commercial fitness centers to exercise. If one is available to you, you will be far better off to avail yourself of one of the facilities that actually specializes in the type of training that we are advocating. You don't have to attend the authors' facilities, there are many throughout North America and throughout the world that specialize in the type of training that we advocate (please see our web site for an up-to-date listing). Given the current environment in a lot of commercial facilities, it might also be wise to try and set up your own training facility in the privacy of your own home.

DISTRACTIONS

QUESTION: Are such things as loud music and mirrors more of a distraction than an aid to training?

ANSWER: Ideally, your workout environment should be one that allows for you to concentrate and that inspires you. To this end, there should be as few distractions as possible that will divert your attention from your purpose. This includes loud music, bright lights, crowds, and mirrors. In the case of mirrors, when you're working out you want to be focusing on producing the highest level of effort that you can and and the deepest level of fatigue in the targeted musculature that you can. And while a lot of trainees have been told that a mirror is a helpful tool for the purpose of observing one's form during exercise, it should be pointed out that form is not a matter of visual input; it's a matter of developing a kinesthetic sense of one's own body. And watching yourself in a mirror (particularly because it is a "mirror image") actually detracts from your form rather than enhancing it. It is far better to internalize what you're feeling and what you're doing rather than relying on a mirror because a mirror really doesn't provide any significant feedback about what is happening with the movement, and may actually distract you from doing the task at hand. What most people are really saying when they say that they like to have a mirror to monitor form is that they like looking at themselves. Unfortunately, looking at yourself can distract you to the point where you simply don't workout as hard as you need to in order to make progress. According to Ken Hutchins, who is one of the few people in the history of exercise science that has looked into the environmental factors (pro and con) of exercise quite thoroughly:

> Mirrors are often haled as an important aid to exercise. Here again, would-be experts like to spew stock notions at face value without investigating their real value. Mirrors are touted as essential to study exercise form. In actuality they are an unnecessary distraction and hindrance in the workout room and a wasteful expense. Try to count the number of exercises where a mirror is actually useful. Remember, that you must conform to the proper neutral positioning of the head and neck and also face the mirror and also view the exercise from the correct angle to criticize the particulars. You will quickly realize that mirrors are almost always worthless for their purported justification. A bodybuilder might say, "I like to watch myself so I can study my form." Since exceedingly few subjects have any notion of what proper form is I must conclude that the second phrase of the sentence can be dropped. If he just admitted that, "I like to look at myself" (and others) I would find his statement more credible. [4]

And this leads us to another potential problem with mirrors involving concentration. Let us envision a scenario wherein one is performing a set of barbell squats. The trainee has shouldered the barbell from the support stands and has stepped back from the stands facing the mirror that is in front of him. He is going to use the mirror now to monitor his form during the exercise; i.e., he's going to try and keep his back straight, his feet spaced apart a certain width and he wants to make sure that he's descending to 90-degrees during the lowering phase of the exercise. As he's attempting to do this, suddenly two people who are several feet behind him but reflected in the mirror become very animated or start play fighting. Several seconds later, a very attractive girl walks by. In both instances, the trainee's attention has been drawn off of the exercise that he's doing. Since squats require a high level of exertion under a heavy load, such momentary lapses in attention can be dangerous. But it's too late; the trainee's attention has been distracted from the performance of the exercise to what is going on behind him and he misjudges his turnaround point in the descent, strains and feels a sudden twinge in his lower back. When checked out later that afternoon by his physician he learns that he has strained a lumbar muscle, which will require that he not workout for perhaps two weeks. All because he placed himself in an environment where he could easily (too easily) be distracted. Particularly in a commercial gym environment where there's lots of movement and people around, a mirror can almost universally be more distracting than helpful to you.

PRIVACY

QUESTION: The owner of the gym I train at gets annoyed if anyone makes a sound while working out. This makes it very hard to give my all to each exercise. Do you encourage silence when you workout or is it okay to make the odd exertional noise?

ANSWER: It's absolutely okay. We don't encourage yelling and screaming as it siphons energy away from the trainee and is not really conducive to proper focus. However, a proper training facility should encourage a hard work ethic. A gym needs to be a place where hard work is recognized and encouraged – not discouraged.

You don't want to be in a very posh commercial establishment that is going to kick you out if you let out a grunt or a groan. The sounds associated with the kind of training we're advocating are *not social*. You have to remember that your purpose in training is to attempt to bring about a biological event; that is, you're trying to bring a stimulus to the body that is severe enough that you're body will make an adaptive response – and the behaviors that attend the type of protocol that is required to achieve this are not social in nature. A proper facility will not tell you to be quiet if let out a scream or snicker at you if you happen to pass wind. These are events that simply attend a high degree of effort. At our facilities we have some clients that are completely stoic when they workout and others that look like Charles Manson. We witness a full spectrum of behaviors that we are accepting and encouraging of. We support whatever you need to do to meet the goal and that needs to be the attitude of the owners of the facility that you workout in.

TEMPERATURE

QUESTION: Is gym temperature an important issue to maximize one's response from exercise?

ANSWER: Yes, the temperature of the workout area is an important consideration for several reasons. One being that if one were to contrast one's performance in an environment that is appropriately cooled and well ventilated with one's performance (in terms of the amount of weight that one can use and the depth of inroad one can produce in terms of weight and Time Under Load) in a warmer unventilated environment, it will always prove to be much better in the environment that's cooler. The reason being that muscular work, like any other work in a closed system, follows the laws of thermodynamics and it is an entropic type of work; that is, it is work that produces a lot of excess heat. A lot of heat is dissipated in the process of fueling muscular contraction and there's also a large degree of friction involved in the movement of muscular contraction. These two factors result in the production of a large amount of internal body heat. And as that temperature rises it will, to a certain extent, enhance one's performance. But after a very small amount of temperature rise, one's performance will actually start to wane because one will start to accumulate internal heat faster than one can dissipate it. Ideally, one would want to train one's muscles in an environment where that heat can be lost easily to the environment through conduction and convection. Conduction is your body directly in contact with cool surfaces, so the temperature in the gym should be cool enough that when you sit on the Naugahyde covered pads of the equipment the direct contact of this ought to feel cold to you, thus producing a gradient that moves from your body onto the equipment that encourages heat loss. And by convection we're talking about heat loss through the air because the surrounding air should be cooler than your body. And this gradient needs to be fairly wide for this to occur in an efficient manner because by the time that one's body has to resort to an evaporative cooling mechanism under this type of exercise, one is already getting to the point where one's performance is going to precipitously drop off.

A COOL WAY TO TRAIN

Ken Hutchins told me that during an osteoporosis research project that he conducted with Arthur Jones back in 1983 or so, that they had an air conditioner that went on the fritz. And just before the air conditioner broke down it began dumping Freon and the training area became really, really cold. And this went on for several days in a row, pushing the temperature in the training area down to 60 degrees and below, but they just pushed on anyway. And what they found was that on the days when the gym temperature was cooler, the performance of the subjects in the study disproportionately improved. So they started experimenting with it and they found that keeping the temperature in the sixties – somewhere between 61 and 68-degrees – with fans blowing on the subjects to increase the convectional heat loss -- resulted in people being able to go to failure with a particular load in a longer period of time, which produced a deeper level of inroad, and, thus, a more potent stimulus. So a cool environment is very conductive to achieving the stimulus that we're after.

-- Doug McGuff, MD

"NO SWEAT" WORKOUTS

QUESTION: I'm skeptical about "not sweating" when I workout. How can I have a productive workout if I don't break a sweat?

ANSWER: As surprising as this may sound to some, there is really no benefit to be had from sweating. People that wear sauna suits or too much clothing while working out often do so in the belief that they will "sweat off" fat – which is simply erroneous thinking. Body fat is roughly 5 to 20 percent water by weight. The fluids that are lost from perspiration come from the blood volume and muscle tissue, not from body fat. What's more, the excess water loss will only hinder fat loss due to the obstruction of muscle function. Once the muscles become dehydrated, their ability to perform work is significantly diminished. In Doug McGuff's facility of 1,200 square feet, he has installed an air conditioner that's big enough to cool a Wal-Mart. And on an August day when it's 102-degrees outside it's only 61-degrees in Doug's facility and there's condensation on the windows because of it.. And in the wintertime it's still 61-degrees. His trainers are dressed in dress slacks, shirt and tie and most of them wear a t-shirt under their dress shirts in the summertime and in the wintertime they'll be wearing either long johns underneath or a sweater over top of their shirts. When his clients start to workout they've got goose bumps, but when they finish their workout the temperature feels perfect to them – but there's not a drop of sweat on them. They literally "don't break a sweat" in Doug's facility. And that is good from his clients' standpoint because they can walk in from their business day, and they can do their workout, get dressed and leave – and they can be door-to-door in 20-minutes without getting all sweaty and dirty. When you think of a person who has to drive 30-minutes to their commercial gym, change clothes, workout, get all sweaty, take a shower, get changed again, drive 30-minutes back to where they work, the amount of time that Doug saves his clients by applying this knowledge of environmental temperature is enormous. He has clients that will arrive at his facility in their dress clothes;

they'll remove their belts, their shirts and their ties, take their dress shoes off and workout in their socks. They'll go through their workout, throw their stuff back on and then head back to work – and they're making better progress than their counterparts who are getting sweaty for an hour or so in a commercial gym. So, the old notion that you have to "break a sweat" in order to have a proper and productive workout is simply wrong. Sweating is simply a mechanism to dissipate the excess heat produced by your body during exertion. There is no rule or law as to how that heat is dissipated, but it takes significant energy that could otherwise be spent on producing more inroad and fatigue to break a sweat. A lot of blood flow has to be diverted to the skin in order to be able to accomplish this; a lot of energy and adrenaline is spent in activating the sweat glands in order for the body to produce sweat. If that adrenaline was instead used to cleave glycogen and keep the inroading process going longer, and to activate hormone sensitive lipase to circulate free fatty acids to keep the process going longer, then all the better. So instead of wasting adrenaline on activating sweat glands to try to keep you cool and maintain thermogenic homeostasis, if you can lose that heat by conduction and convection, you can spare the adrenaline for cleaving more glycogen and activating hormone sensitive lipase to provide the fuel necessary to continue to inroad deeper and thus provide a better stimulus for positive adaptive change from exercise.

A FAN OF BETTER WORKOUTS

In addition to keeping the temperature in my facility at 61-degrees, every machine that I have in the gym has a fan stationed in front of it. So you're sitting in the machine in an environment that is deliberately set at 61-degrees with a fan blowing directly on you that is set at "high." I mean, people's shorts and t-shirts are flapping in the breeze. And a lot of people will initially hate it, particularly when you're first starting your workout and you're initially chilly, but what they find is if we ever have a day where the air conditioner isn't working or it's a little warmer than usual (such as if it's a really hot day and we can't get the temperature down to 61-degrees for whatever reason), the clients will complain about it because they can really notice the difference. Until you've experienced this it is truly astounding the difference between working out in a properly cooled exercise environment and one that is not properly cooled. The difference between working out at 61-degrees versus 72-degrees is unbelievable. I mean when I'm out of town and have to train at a commercial facility that doesn't have proper temperature control in their workout area, it is unbelievable what a difference it makes in terms of the intensity that you can bring to your workout.

-- Doug McGuff, MD

WORKING WITH A TRAINER

QUESTION: A lot of what goes into having a good workout is psychological. In particular, do you find that when a client knows that someone is present supervising his workout that it inspires him train harder?

ANSWER: This is referred to in the scientific literature as the "Hawthorne Effect," in reference to a study that was conducted on worker productivity in factories during the 1950s. The experimenters found that just the act of observing the workers increased their productivity. Likewise, just the act of having someone supervise your workout will increase your workout intensity markedly.

A NON-THREATFUL ENVIORNMENT

QUESTION: Are you in favor (as many Superslow ^{TM} trainers seem to be) of having a trainer dressed in dress shirt and slacks when they train clients – and, if so, why?

ANSWER: While many personal training centers downplay the importance of having their trainers dress professionally (i.e., wearing dress pants, shirt and tie), believing that if an individual is properly focused on his workout, it shouldn't matter what anybody else is wearing, there is a reason why a facility should have their trainers dress markedly different than the way that their clients are dressed when they workout. A dress code for trainers isn't simply something that makes trainers look good; it is a means by which they can keep the focus of the client solely on the workout itself. It is a means by which they are viewed by the trainee as authoritative but "non threatening" to (and "non competitive" with) the trainee's aspirations. A trainer's authority in getting someone to push himself beyond his comfort zone is predicated on his authority with the trainee. But it is also predicated upon the assumption that the trainer is doing nothing to "compete" with the trainee or to dominate them. There have been studies [5, 6, 7, 8] that examined the serum testosterone levels present in people that were either winning or losing a game and found that winners (and even the fans of the winners) produced significantly higher levels of serum testosterone than did the losers (and the fans of the losers). Similarly, if a well-conditioned, muscular instructor dressed in workout attire such that his musculature is visible will appear more dominant to the client that is working out. And that psychological challenge wherein the client feels defeated will negatively influence the intensity that he can bring to the exercise he is performing. That sort of display does not provide inspiration to a client, it instead provides *intimidation*. It's important that the trainer understands that the client is the one working out – not the trainer. The instructor is there to instruct, not to workout, and so he should not dress as though he was going to workout. The more professionally the instructor dresses, the more authority he will carry without being threatening in a way that is going to inhibit the client from performing maximally. Hence, the authors' tendency to prefer more formal attire – dress slacks, dress shirt, tie, etc. – because such dress disguises any potential competition between the trainer and the client and also gives the instructor an air of professionalism and authority such that he can safely push the client in a way that is non-threatening.

EQUIPMENT SET UP

QUESTION: How would you recommend that the equipment be set up in a training facility in order to maximize concentration and effort?

ANSWER: We prefer the equipment to be facing a blank wall and/or to face the exterior of the workout environment rather than its interior. This prevents someone who may be traversing through the workout environment from looking at the trainee while he or she is working out. This ensures that no one is making direct eye contact with the trainee, no one is getting in his or her line of vision to distract them, and, thus, prevents situations from occurring where, in the middle of a high exertion set, a social nicety becomes necessary, such as acknowledging someone or saying, "Hello." These are events that have their time and place, but during the workout is neither. When someone is working out that workout should be the totality of his or her focus and the training environment should take this into account and be set up so that there is as little distraction as possible.

LOUD MUSIC

QUESTION: What's wrong with having loud music playing when you workout? I always feel more motivated when I have loud rock music playing in the gym.

ANSWER: We've learned that the gym should be quiet for optimal concentration. Ideally, there should be no music playing during the workout. And under this same category we do not allow our instructors to carry cell phones around with them when training clients. The trainer's focus needs to be on the client during the client's workout – and nothing else. We concede that for some people music can be inspiring and it can serve to motivate them, but even with this concession it remains a distraction. Often the tempo of the music being played can psychologically or subconsciously set the tempo for the exercise movement that one is performing and very often the two are out of synch.

CHILDREN IN THE WORKOUT ENVIRONMENT

QUESTION: I'm a single mother. If I'm going to workout, I have to be able to bring my child with me to the gym, *as I do not have a babysitter. Will this impede my workout efforts?*

ANSWER: While we understand that you will need to bring your children with you to the gym, we would advise against bringing your children directly into the workout area when you are training. There are those Moms and Dads that have two or three small children and simply have to bring them to the gym with them. But even in such a scenario, select a gym that has a Day Care area that is well supervised or, if it's a smaller center, check to see if the facility has a Pack 'n Play, or Play Pen that the child can be placed in and a television and/or DVD player that will play age-appropriate programs to occupy them during the time of your workout. You should also have the trainer lock the door to the facility during this period of time and put up a "Closed" sign in the window until your workout has concluded and you are reunited with your child (or children) again.

YELLING IS NO ENCOURAGMENT

QUESTION: When you're training a client do you recommend yelling encouragement when he is struggling with his last rep or two – or does this not help?

ANWER: When we train clients we do so using a very calm reassuring tone of voice. We don't bark out exhortations to the client to complete his repetitions in good form. To some extent how much we speak depends upon the client and what works for hm and is something that is discerned over time. But the philosophy we have – and it's the philosophy of *Body By Science* – is to spend time trying to provide the client with an intellectual understanding of what he or she is trying to achieve. And this is very important because every instinct that you have rebels and tries to find a way around the stimulus of deep inroading. Consequently, in order for a workout to result in optimal stimulation to one's muscles one first has to have a deep intellectual understanding of what the goal of the workout process is.

AN INTELLECTUAL APPROACH

QUESTION: Do you take the time to explain to the client all of the "whys" and "wherefores" of the Body By Science approach prior to their working out, or is client education not as important as trainer education?

ANSWER: Both are important. A good trainer should take the time to explain the importance of why the client needs to perform very hard work, so that everyone involved in the process has an understanding of what the goal is. This requires an intellectual approach and an intellectual approach is a calm, methodical, stern and stoic approach. We don't use ammonia caps, we don't scream and yell. Instead, we act like people that are on a mission and we do what we need to do to accomplish that mission but without the drama. A good trainer understands that his client needs to concentrate in order to be able to work as hard as possible. When a trainer speaks to a client it should only be to provide important instructional details. And if he doesn't have important instructional details to impart, then he should keep quiet so that the client can better concentrate. And if during the course of your workout you can converse with your trainer about your weekend, or what your kids are doing, or about politics, then you're not working out hard enough. If you can speak, something's wrong. Remember, you're going to a workout facility for one thing – to workout. It's not a social visit.

COLOGNE PROBLEMS

QUESTION: My trainer reeks of cologne when he trains me. I almost gag on it. Do you have any policies for your trainers regarding wearing colognes or perfumes or am I simply being too sensitive?

ANSWER: No, you're not being too sensitive. We recommend that whoever is training you not be wearing powerful colognes or deodorants. If you're polishing off a set of Leg Presses at the end of your workout and you're in metabolic hell, the smell of someone's perfume might be just the thing that pushes you over the edge and makes you sick.

PAYING A PERSONAL TRAINER

QUESTION: Why should I pay a personal trainer to work me out? What's the advantage?

ANSWER: Well, that will depend upon what value you place on your time. As owners of personal training centers, we believe that our clients' time is valuable. And as such, we don't encourage anyone to waste what little he or she has of it. For that matter, the time of your trainer is also valuable. Ideally, you should be looking to enter into a value-for-value exchange with a competent trainer in which your body is strengthened and your fitness goals are pursued under the supervision of someone that is paid the appropriate market value for his or her services and who will provide you with the facility, equipment and expertise necessary to realize your goals without wasting your valuable time. Many commercial fitness centers will charge their members a membership fee and up to $100 a workout for a client to have a personal trainer with them. By contrast, most high-intensity personal training centers charge in the neighborhood of $35 to $50 a session, which is quite reasonable by contrast. Some people make the mistake of attempting to assess value based upon the amount of *time* that a trainer spends with them, when what they should be predicating their pricing on is *results*. Clients also need to calculate into their decision not only what they are paying to have access to a facility and trainer, but also the additional costs that they will be absorbing as a result of being out of their productive loop for the period of time that they are working out. After all, during the period of time that they will be working out they won't be working at their job (and, thus, not making money) and they also can't be at home enjoying "off" time, which likewise has a value that should be the equivalent of one's hourly wage. Let's assume that there are two executives that want to become stronger for fitness reasons. Both executives earn 100 dollars an hour. The first executive goes the more conventional route; he goes to the gym three days a week for an hour a session under the watchful eye of an instructor who charges him $100 an hour, plus a membership fee at the facility of $50 a month. Since he's out of the work loop for one hour to meet his fitness goals, three days a week, he's not only out the $300 a week (plus membership dues) for the cost of the workouts, but he also has to count the $300 that he lost by not working and the value of that same $300 that he could have been spending with his wife and children. This alone has taken at least $900 of value-based time out of his income. Now, by contrast, if another executive who makes 100 dollars an hour goes to a personal training center owned by someone who has the best equipment, the proper workout environment and the instructional experience to get him comparable or better results in 12-minutes once a week for a fee of $35 to $50, which executive comes out of the experience ahead? If you said, "the first executive," you need to think again. Look at the facts: the second executive will obtain the same or better results and he or she is going to have 2 hours of his or her time returned, which is valued at $100 an hour (x 2 because he or she is going to get back either work time or family time -- or both). In other words, the second executive will have $230 to $460 worth of his or her valuable time back for the expenditure of $35 or $50. However, this is based on the assumption that the results are going to be equivalent from both the commercial fitness center approach of three days per week for an hour each session and the 20-minutes once a week approach of a high-intensity training center. But what typically happens in the commercial fitness center with training that is either self-directed or directed by an uniformed instructor is that the results are *not* equivalent. The trainee, then, ends up spending all that time for a return of little or no results (or in many cases negative results). It should be true that you get what you pay for, but in the case of most commercial fitness centers it isn't.

PART FIVE: NUTRITION

NUTRITIONAL GENETICS

QUESTION: I like that Body By Science is based upon evolutionary biology. Can you elaborate on what this means in terms of our nutritional requirements?

ANSWER: To begin with, it means that humans are amazingly adaptive. In terms of our physical capacity, if called upon we can swim for miles, walk for days, and bring down predatory prey much larger than ourselves. Much of how our body responds and performs must be viewed within the context of survival, as many of the things mentioned we evolved a capacity to do in an environment that required us to do them *periodically*. However, in terms of modern day exercise, these are not things that we should choose to do. After all, while it's true that our ancestors walked for tens of thousands of miles they did not do so for exercise. They did so because they had to in order to search for food (energy). And, as a result of these types of activities (and as we indicated in *Body By Science*), most of them died with bone-crippling osteoarthritis and enjoyed a much shorter life expectancy than we do presently. And while our ancestors experienced brief periods of "fight or flight" behavior (i.e., behavior that tapped higher order motor units) throughout their lives, these events occurred very infrequently and thus led to our metabolic health requirements being established. And over eons the human genotype evolved in a manner that grants us tremendous plasticity. We could adapt while other lesser animals could not, which is why we are here today and those other species have exited the planet (roughly 98 percent of all animal forms that have lived on this earth are now extinct). From a nutritional standpoint, it's important to recall that our genome evolved from a hunter/gatherer background during times when food energy was in short supply. Consequently our bodies became very resourceful, as they would have to be in order to make use of whatever foodstuffs we had available in order to convert such foodstuffs into the nutrients or materials necessary for us to survive and to be healthy enough to adapt to the vicissitudes of life in an often-uncooperative environment. As a consequence of this, the human animal evolved as an omnivore, capable of eating almost anything. We have the metabolic machinery to take whatever we shove down our necks and turn it into almost anything that we require. If you refer to the metabolic diagrams accompanying Chapters 2 and 9 in *Body By Science*, you will see this fact written out in long form. Indeed, the fate of what you eat does not have so much to do with *what* you eat, as it has to do with the underlying demands your body must meet. As a result, if there is a strong stimulus for muscle growth, your body will take whatever nutrients it gets and turns them into the required substrates. For instance, if your body takes in carbohydrates when it needs protein synthesis, it will take the caloric energy from the carbohydrate and use it for synthesizing new proteins. If you eat protein and your body needs to replenish its glycogen stores, it can take the amino acids and synthesize them back to pyruvate and then to glucose through a process called gluconeogenesis. The glucose thus produced can then be stored as glycogen. Consequently, most people's diets possess an abundant source of substrate for muscle growth, if stimulated, to occur. At our personal training facilities there are physicians, accountants, financial advisors, business owners, factory workers, and professional educators who have never picked up a bodybuilding magazine, have never heard of the "fat burning" power of herbal supplements, don't drink green tea, don't consume "energy" drinks and do not take supplemental protein and yet are showing progress that most bodybuilding enthusiasts would kill for. If you want the most bang for your nutritional dollar, then provide your body with a high-intensity training stimulus that will shunt your nutritional substrate in the desired direction. If the stimulus is of high-intensity and your recovery period is adequate, you could almost make good progress on a diet of Skittles ® (note that we say "almost" for reasons to follow). And this is as it must be, owing to the fact that our ancestors (particularly in hunter/gatherer times) didn't have the luxury of controlling the seasons during which particular herbs and plant sources of vitamins and minerals blossomed. Consequently, they most certainly didn't have the luxury of being able to sit down to a completely balanced three-to-five-course meal three times a day, seven-days a week. They might have been lucky enough to eat leafy green vegetables such as lettuce and spinach one day and then not be able to consume them again for two-to-three weeks. Meat was preferred because its fat content yielded more calories per gram (9 calories per gram of fat versus 4 calories per gram of either carbohydrate or protein), but a great deal more calories were required in expenditure in order to obtain it – and it might not return to the diet for another month or so, depending upon what animals were present in the environment that our ancestors were occupying. So our nutritional value was placed at the expediency of the moment; i.e., whatever was around that was edible was consumed, and our ancestors did so in order to survive; i.e., to take in enough energy to keep their physiological machines running until they encountered more fuel again. The ability to know that our body has specific nutritional needs and knowing what these needs are and how they apply to our health – as opposed to merely pursuing food out of hunger -- most certainly represents an advancement and "evolution" in terms of our nutritional knowledge that is light years beyond that of our hunter-gatherer ancestors. Moreover, with this knowledge, we have set up food centers that make it far easier for us in present day to obtain the necessary foodstuffs to enhance our body's health. Our ancestors had to walk for miles in order to cover terrain to look for plants to eat, and to systemically bring down large game. These were activities that were highly dangerous. By contrast, we merely have to stroll down the aisle at our local supermarket to do our present day hunting and gathering. However, as our knowledge about nutrition and its effect on the human body has increased, we have also come to learn that although our genome has evolved a mechanism whereby we can eat almost anything, this does not mean that this is absolutely the best way to proceed nutritionally, anymore than the fact that our ancestors walked for miles in the pursuit of food and ultimately developed bone crippling osteoarthritis from having done so is the best way to proceed to achieve our fitness goals.

A WELL-BALANCED DIET

QUESTION: *You advocate consuming a well-balanced diet. What exactly is this?*

ANSWER: Nutritional scientists have divided foods into four groups based upon their role in the diet and their nutritive value. According to them a well-balanced diet includes several servings from each group every day. A "serving," incidentally, is the average, such as 3-ounces of meat, and does not include sauces or gravies. Here is how it breaks down:

- Lean Meats – meat, fish, poultry, eggs, nuts and beans (2 or more servings a day)
- Fruits and Vegetables (4 or more servings a day)
- Milk and Dairy Products (2 or more glasses of milk or servings of cheese or butter)
- Cereals and Grains (4 or more servings. Please note, we are in disagreement with this last category for reasons to follow)

The nutrients contained in a well-balanced diet include the three macronutrients of protein, fat and carbohydrate. Carbohydrates, while not without risk, are the body's main source of fuel. They're stored in the muscles and liver in the form of energy-giving glycogen. Fats are stored in the muscles, under the skin, and around body organs and are the second-best source of energy. Protein, although it enjoys a special status in the fitness and bodybuilding world, is a poor energy provider at any time and the body has no way of storing it.

WATER

QUESTION: *I read in your chapter on fat loss of the importance of water to optimize one's hormonal response to exercise. How important is water to the non-dieting trainee?*

ANSWER: Water is without question the most important of all the nutrients as we can live for some time without carbohydrates, fat and protein, but only a few days without water. The importance of water is obvious when you consider that the body is 60 percent water. Water not only contains valuable minerals, but it also acts as a lubricator, a shock absorber between cells, a digestion aid, and is the body's primary means of cooling, performing the essential job of maintaining the body's normal temperature. In the course of an average day the average human body loses water steadily, though up to 50 percent of this loss goes largely unseen. On a hot day it's not uncommon to lose five to eight quarts of fluid that must then be replaced either by drinking liquids or through food. A surprising amount of seemingly solid food contains a high percentage of water. Meats, for instance, can be as much as 50 percent water and most fruits and vegetables can be as high as 79 percent.

FATS

QUESTION: What are fats?

ANSWER: Fats, or lipids, are chemical compounds that don't dissolve in water. Roughly 98 percent of most fats are called triglycerides of which some are saturated and come from animals and some are unsaturated and come from plants.

PROTEIN

QUESTION: What is protein exactly?

ANSWER: Protein is organic material that, next to water, is the primary structural material of the body's cells and tissues. There are roughly 20 amino acids in protein and at least nine of these (the "essential" amino acids) have to be obtained from the daily diet. But just as the body doesn't care where it gets its glucose, it likewise isn't concerned about the source of its protein. In other words, from the body's vantage point the protein contained in beans is just as good as the protein contained in meat. Protein is absolutely essential for the growth and repair of the body's tissues but it has yet to be proven that more than enough of any essential element of nutrition is better for the body than merely enough. The average adult needs about 70 grams of protein per day for normal growth and development., which roughly translates into 9-ounces of broiled hamburger.

CARBOHYDRATES

QUESTION: *What are carbohydrates?*

ANSWER: Carbohydrates are chemical compounds of sugar, starches and cellulose (fiber) containing carbon, hydrogen, and oxygen. The most important carbohydrate is glucose, the body's primary energy source. The sugar molecules in food are called monosaccharides (individual molecules), disaccharides (pairs of molecules) and polysaccharides (three or more molecules). The body, however, can only absorb monosaccharides so it chemically breaks down the di- and poly saccharides into monosaccharides, which find their way to the liver, where fructose and galactose are converted to glucose and used for energy. Sugar, because it contains readily usable glucose, is absorbed into the bloodstream very quickly. By contrast, starches need to be broken down and are therefore absorbed slowly. The original source of the glucose doesn't matter to your body (i.e., it can convert the carbohydrate found in ice cream or a potato into glucose), as, in short, to your bloodstream glucose is glucose. As a source of energy, however, refined sugars are a poor choice. They are absorbed immediately and this will result in spikes in glucose levels, which, as we'll soon see, can lead to a host of problems. By contrast, the more unrefined sugars, such as those found in potatoes and peas, take longer for the body to process and thus provide a slower rise in glucose levels. Typically there is less than a quarter of an ounce of glucose available in the bloodstream at any one time, but the body stores an additional 12-ounces of glucose in the heart and muscle tissue. This reserve energy is used on site during muscular activity.

ESSENTIAL MACRONUTRIENTS

QUESTION: What are essential nutrients (i.e., nutrients that the body actually needs)?

ANSWER: By "essential" we mean nutrients that can only be acquired through the diet and that cannot be synthesized *de novo* in the body.

ESSENTIAL PROTEINS

QUESTION: Are there essential proteins (i.e., amino acids) that should be present in our diet?

ANSWER: Yes. Amino acids such as isoleucine, leucine, lysine, threonine, tryptophan, methionine, histidine, valine are the "Big 8" considered to be "essential."

ESSENTIAL FATS

QUESTION: Are there any essential fats that should be present in our diet?

ANSWER: Yes. Essential fatty acids such as linolenic acid and arachidonic acid can only be acquired from the diet.

ESSENTIAL CARBOHYDATES

QUESTION: Are there any essential carbohydrates that should be present in our diet?

ANSWER: The answer, surprisingly, is no. The reality is that there isn't *any* carbohydrate that needs to be acquired from the diet that cannot be synthesized from something else. Indeed, if you look at hunter-gatherer civilizations that are still on-going and if you look at the anthropological data surrounding the nutritional consumption of our ancestors, you will find that carbohydrate is not only the least abundant foodstuff that we can acquire in terms of nutrient density, but it is also not essential to the diet for the simple fact that glucose (the final common substrate of carbohydrate) can be synthesized through the metabolic process of gluconeogenesis from the proteins that we eat.

PROBLEMS WITH HIGH CARBOHYDRATE INTAKE

QUESTION: But since we evolved as omnivores that can turn anything we eat into what we need, why does it matter if we consume a diet that has more carbohydrates or sugars in it?

ANSWER: The fact that we *can* do this doesn't mean that we *should* do this – any more than the fact that we can walk a 100 miles doesn't mean that we should this for exercise. Moreover, the fact that we can do this does not come without significant metabolic and hormonal consequences that can negatively impact our health and our results from exercise. When one looks at hunter-gatherer diets in terms of macronutrient ingestion, the bulk of their diets were made up of protein and fats obtained through hunted meats and other foodstuffs. [1,2] Any carbohydrate that could be found was such as grew wild, which meant that it was high in fiber, [3] not calorie-dense, and, thus, when it was converted into glucose it was done so slowly and released into the bloodstream slowly as well. The slow rise in glucose levels served to keep the hunter-gatherer's serum insulin levels relatively low, which served an important function in the health of the organism. [4, 5] Having a high rise in insulin levels is undesirable for several reasons, one of which is that insulin, as a hormone, trumps almost every other hormone that opposes it – including hormones that allow us to release stored energy (body fat). Hormones such as testosterone, growth hormone, and glucagons are hormones that are strongly involved in releasing energy from the body from any source depot – whether glycogen or bodyfat. Insulin, if present in high enough levels, will effectively override or trump these other hormones, thus preventing mobilization of these energy sources. High insulin levels, then, will inhibit the body's ability to activate hormones and enzymes such as hormone-sensitive lipase that act together to cleave glycogen and mobilize energy substrate that enable the body to lose bodyfat. With obesity being such a huge modern problem, consuming a type of diet that results in a raising of one's serum insulin levels– even in the face of a caloric deficit diet – the body's ability to control its skyrocketing insulin levels becomes increasingly important. A high-intensity exercise program goes a long way in helping with this process by maintaining insulin sensitivity as a direct effect of emptying the muscles of their glycogen and also activating hormone-sensitive lipase, which allows us to mobilize fatty acids. But even then, it is very easy to out-eat an exercise program or undo its effects by eating too much of the wrong foods.

NUTRITION: INDUSTRY VERSUS REALITY

QUESTION: Why is your nutritional paradigm not generally embraced by the bodybuilding and fitness industries?

ANSWER: Largely because the nutritional paradigm that has been put forth by the fitness and bodybuilding industry is heavily predicated on the sale of supplements, which has very little basis in reality. If having to prepare special meals of egg whites and oatmeal that are then carried around with the trainee throughout the day in little Tupperware containers to be consumed at specific intervals several times a day were necessary for optimal health, then we would never have survived as a species. Not only is the typical fitness industry diet not necessary, it's not desirable as it actually serves to produce a type of nutrition that drives insulin levels higher, which is highly counterproductive as it prevents our bodies from being able to produce an optimal response to the exercise stimulus. By contrast, a well-balanced diet that relies on whole natural foods as much possible, that includes lean meats, fruits and vegetables is both necessary and desirable. Despite what we've indicated about carbohydrates, we are not "anti-carbohydrate" by any means, and we do not recommend that one restrict their intake of carbohydrate as a macronutrient group. Instead, we recommend that the carbohydrate that one consumes be in the form of fibrous fruits and vegetables. The carbohydrate sources that one should choose to avoid are those that are grain-based and/or refined in nature. And these two things go hand in hand, as grain (the seed head in plants) cannot be digested in humans. The only way that grain can be digested is if it is altered in form by first being ground into flour and then mixed with other ingredients to produce a matrix that can then be cooked and consumed. And even this process can be problematic, as in the process of converting the seed head of plants into something that is digestible by humans, carbohydrate is released from the fibrous matrix that it's normally encased in, with the result that an inordinately large amount of glucose enters the circulation very quickly, rising to high levels in a sudden fashion that requires large pulses of insulin to be present in order to metabolize the glucose. This process results in a rapid storage of glycogen in the muscle, thus capping off of the glycogen stores in the muscle, and producing an overall loss of insulin sensitivity and, therefore, chronically elevated levels of insulin.

MORE PROBLEMS WITH GRAIN-BASED FOOD

QUESTION: Are there any other problems that attend eating grain-based foods?

ANSWER: Yes, particularly with the fatty acids that are contained within them. If, for instance, one is consuming beef that has been grass fed as opposed to grain fed, one will be eating in such a way that one's carbohydrate content is containing more Omega 3 fatty acids, which is a fatty acid profile that actually is the hormonal precursor of the anti-inflammatory prostaglandin and leukotriene. [6] However, if you're eating beef that has been consuming grain sources, these grains will contain a much higher content of Omega 6, Omega 9 and other types of fatty acids that are the metabolic precursors of the inflammatory prostaglandin and leukotrienes.[7] The Omega 3s, in other words, are all series 3 prostaglandins that are anti-inflammatory; the Omega 6s and others are precursors to the series 6 prostaglandins, which *are* inflammatory and the balance between these two will determine to a large extent the degree of systemic inflammation that your body will have to deal with. Consequently, eating foodstuffs (and even food that eats foodstuffs) that fall outside of our hunter-gatherer range produces not just increased insulin levels, it also produces other negative side effects in terms of systemic inflammation. [8]

CARBS ARE NOT VILLAINS

QUESTION: So are you saying that carbohydrates – as a food group – are bad for us?

ANSWER: No, we're simply saying that for health purposes you are better served obtaining them from fruits and vegetables, rather than from bread, flour and sugar. These latter sources of carbohydrate are converted to glucose in the bloodstream much more quickly as their fiber density is minimal to non-existent, resulting in higher glucose levels, and this results in the body defending itself by producing higher levels of insulin. And the hormonal consequence of this can be very counterproductive to the body on multiple levels. Carbohydrate ingested from fruit and vegetable sources provide not only glucose, but also vitamins and minerals, which are contained in the phytochemicals of the fruits and vegetables themselves. The term "phyto" comes from the Greek word that means "plant," and the phytochemicals are usually related to plant pigments. Consequently, the fruits and vegetables that are bright colors, such as yellow, orange, red, green, blue, and purple, generally contain the greatest quantity of phytochemicals, and, as a result, the most nutrients. Sugar, by contrast, can be quickly converted to glucose, but it contains "zero" vitamins and minerals.

VITAMINS

QUESTION: *Are you in favor of taking vitamin supplements?*

ANSWER: What one needs to keep in mind about vitamins is that they are co-factors that produce their benefit in the context of the food matrix in which they're contained. Consequently, when they are removed from this context they may no longer be effective. If, for instance, you wish to obtain the anti-oxidant benefit of resveratrol then it would be better to drink red wine or eat muskadine grapes – rather than to obtain it from a supplement. In other words, it's better to obtain this element in the context of the whole food in which it is contained. A lot of people who fancy themselves anti-aging experts advocate incredibly complex (up to 100 vitamin pills a day!) supplement regimens that are completely unnecessary. If you're eating a natural whole foods diet, then you're going to be much better off than by trying to cobble together a proper diet through some sort of supplement regimen.

NUTRIENT COMPETITION

QUESTION: *I'm still not clear as to why it's so important to watch our intake of refined carbohydrates and grain-based foods. What am I missing here?*

ANSWER: Perhaps you're missing the context that human metabolism is not a centralized totalitarian-style "command and control" process. Indeed, all of the tissues in the body will only cooperate in a harmonious homeostatic mechanism under certain circumstances. As a result of the fact that all of our bodily tissues delineate from a cell line that has different potentials, these tissues, then, depending upon the stimulus each receives during their development, will develop into different things. And not only do they interact with each other in a way that is cooperative to the whole organism, but this occurs within a context that's more like a market; that is, they compete with each other for the resources that are brought into the body. This means that muscle tissue and fat tissue don't exist to harmoniously support each other, they exist in an environment that is competitive. And while your body can take anything you eat and turn it into what you need, that is true because if it weren't true, probably eight percent of our population would be dead based upon the type of diets that they're following. Again, just because your body has this capability, it doesn't follow that this is a desirable or preferable capacity to engage on a continuous basis. In other words, the fact that a capacity exists does not give us grounds to abuse it on an on-going basis. As with exercise, just because the body can adapt doesn't mean that it possesses and infinite capacity for adaptation and one can quickly run it into the ground with too much exercise. Similarly with nutrition, if you overload the system with a particular macronutrient such as carbohydrate (or even protein), it can adapt to it up to a certain point. Beyond this point, however, one can run into trouble.

PROTEIN PROBLEMS

QUESTION: What is wrong with supplementing our diet with large amounts of protein? After all, when you workout with weights your goal is to build muscle and protein is part of muscle.

ANSWER: Excessive protein intake will cause one's urine to change color (the nitrogen makes urine a darker shade of yellow) and also increase urination frequency. This results in a rate of fluid loss that can induce a state of dehydration, which has the capacity to significantly impede performance, as well as place an inordinate strain on one's kidneys. According to a report in the International Journal of Sports Nutrition:

> There can be a "four to fivefold increase in urine volume" in some individuals consuming excessive protein intakes (greater than 2.0 g per 2.2 lb body weight.) [9]

It is simply not necessary to overdose on any one of the macronutrients to the exclusion or the diminishment of others. If, for instance, carbohydrate intake is insufficient in one's diet, one's body will actually take an amino acid (alinine) and break it down in the liver and convert it to glucose. So your body does require sufficient carbohydrate in order to create sufficient glucose or else it will break down your muscle tissue to create its own. Indeed, almost 100 percent of the fuel for brain and nervous system function is derived from glucose. And while it can be produced by other substrates, the body's preferred nutrient for glucose manufacturing is carbohydrate which is why carbohydrates are referred to as "protein sparing," as they "spare" protein from being used as a fuel source, allowing it to be employed in its primary function for growth and repair. There simply exists no need to take additional amino acids or protein over and above one's diet in order to "help" with the muscle building process. In fact, not taking in enough protein results in a process of tapping an essential acid out of the musculature, and this is something that can prove to have long-term androgenic effects on the body. The body's response to tapping out amino acids and then replacing them produces a hormonal environment in which growth hormone and glucagon (among others) actually enhance the production of muscle tissue. To this extent, the tapping an amino acid out of the musculature is akin to a workout; i.e., there has to be some breakdown, some loss, to occur in order for super-compensation (growth) to occur. In the same way that glycogen can super-compensate when tapped out of a muscle, the mobilization of the glucogenic amino acids out of the muscle cell substrate produces a similar sort of effect. In other words, your body's ability to make this conversion is not a decidedly undesirable occurrence. The point to keep in mind about macronutrients – any macronutrient – is to make every effort to obtain them from food sources that have some sort of evolutionary background to them, as opposed to sources that have been refined. And this applies to protein sources as well as carbohydrate sources. If one obtains one's protein from a powder rather than food, it also can result in a rapid absorption, and a rapid production of gluconeogenesis, triggering an excess insulin response in much the same manner as if you had consumed flour or table sugar.

THE BIG LIE

QUESTION: So taking a "super" supplement blend will NOT contribute to making me "super" healthy?

ANSWER: Correct. The big danger is in the big lie; i.e., that people can obtain a "super diet" that will then result in "super health." Such a notion strikes the authors as the equivalent of trying to play pool with a rope rather than a cue stick. In either scenario you cannot force the situation from the supply side of things. Any attempt to obtain super nutrition to drive the process from the supply side only results in a hormonal response that is counter productive, as any form of over nutrition is going to result in elevated insulin levels, which is going to result in chronic inflammation, and a metabolism that will produce excess oxidative damage and compromise one's recovery ability.

THE WELL BALANCED DIET REVISITED

QUESTION: So what nutrient ratios would you recommend in order to obtain a well-balanced diet?

ANSWER: We don't recommend that the reader break his or her diet into macronutrient ratios (such as specific percentages of carbohydrates, protein and fat), and not because such ratios may be improper, but rather because then people tend to look at food labels or consult diet books while attempting to comprise everything they eat within the context of such a balance. This results in overcomplicating the process and can lead to compliance problems over time. The reality is that if we consume natural foodstuffs we can tolerate different macronutrient mixes that are widely variant. And this is how it should be, given that we evolved as a species that lived in an environment of four seasons and the changing seasons drastically altered the macronutrient mix that we, as hunter-gatherer animals, might encounter. Consequently, one can vacillate back and forth between, say, a carbohydrate intake in one's diet that is sometimes as high as 60 to 70 percent, and at times as low as 0 to 10 percent, without ill consequence. The more important point is that we obtain our food from natural, whole food sources such as various types of lean meats, fruits and vegetables, such as we had available to us as hunter-gatherers. The concept of having a specific mix of macronutrients is predicated on trying to manage an improper intake of foodstuffs more than it is predicated on any actual science that supports one percentage mixture being better than another.

A SAMPLE DIET

QUESTION: Can you provide an example of what a proper sample diet might look like?

ANSWER: A sample diet might consist of a breakfast consisting of slices of cantaloupe, grapefruit, grapes and apples one morning (which would be 100 percent carbohydrate), a grass-fed beef burger patty, green salad and stick of cheese for lunch (which would contain a large protein emphasis), and a dinner consisting of turkey, broccoli and one or two other vegetables. This could be changed from time to time to emphasize different macronutrients, but such a diet would be healthy and contribute to the overall health of the organism.

TRAINING AND DIETARY LATITUDE

QUESTION: Does high-intensity training, owing to the fact that it empties a considerable amount of glycogen out of our muscles, allow the trainee a lot more latitude in terms of his everyday dietary behavior?

ANSWER: Absolutely. Despite our best efforts to stick within the parameters of a hunter-gatherer type of diet, we recognize that there will be times when we slip up and have, say, pizza or ice cream from time to time. The consequences of this for someone who is performing the type of exercise we advocate, providing such occurrences are infrequent, will be next to nil, which makes the long-term compliance with this type of dietary philosophy much easier to achieve. And this is important owing to the inescapable fact that one can't just cut oneself off from the world. Somewhere, sometime, you're going to want a donut and the world is not going to stop revolving because of this. There have been periods of years during the authors' lives when their diet was absolutely terrible, but we didn't get fat, or develop diabetes or reduce our insulin sensitivity because of the beneficial effect of the high-intensity training that we engaged in. And when such benefits from training are combined with an eating plan in which people obtain their meat, fruits and vegetables in the form that nature actually delivers them, as opposed to ground up and reconstituted in some other form that's quickly absorbed, digested and results in high spikes of glucose and insulin, one feels better, performs better and body fat is not gained nearly as readily.

FATTY ACIDS

QUESTION: What are your thoughts on fatty acids – what types are best?

ANSWER: The types of fatty acids that we obtain from natural sources such as fish, from naturally obtained fowl, from grass fed beef, contain essential amino acids that not only are essential ingredients for making up the components of cell membranes but are the essential backbones for producing the sex steroids and other hormones that are important to the process that we're trying to achieve. In addition, such a diet also contains sufficient quantity of the type of fatty acids that, when present in the diet and when circulating in the body, serve to up-regulate the enzymes that are necessary and important for fatty acid mobilization. And this is a decided benefit for anyone who's interested in losing bodyfat.

NATURAL FOODS VS HEALTH FOODS

QUESTION: You seem to be in favor of natural foods. What's the difference between natural foods and health foods?

ANSWER: When we speak of "natural" foods please do not confuse this to mean what is popularly termed "health foods." Food scientists and supplement companies will not improve upon what is already offered us by Mother Nature – and we're not coming at this from a "design" standpoint, but rather from an evolved species standpoint. In other words, natural food wasn't designed for us to eat, but rather we evolved to eat the food that was made available to us by nature.

TIME TO EAT

QUESTION: I've heard that you shouldn't eat after 7:00 p.m. and that you should have seven smaller meals a day instead of three bigger ones. What are your thoughts on that?

ANSWER: While some have argued that eating more frequently generates a greater thermic cost of digestion from consuming a greater quantity of smaller meals, the difference between these and three slightly larger meals is nominal. Besides, while we have no knowledge of what your sleep/wake cycle is, based on our lives we have to ask how do you fit seven meals per day in and NOT eat after 7:00 p.m.? If, for instance, it was absolutely necessary that you could only eat carbohydrates before a certain time and proteins and fats before a certain time of the day then we could not have survived as a species because hunter-gatherers ate what they could when it was available – and that's the genotype that we've inherited.

FAT GAIN

QUESTION: *I found what you said about individuals whose nutrient partitioning is such that almost all calorie intake goes to fat storage absolutely fascinating. Can you tell me more about this process?*

ANSWER: Certainly. When your glucose levels are full and, thus, your insulin levels are high, and you continue to eat a lot of refined sugars, then there's only one metabolic destination for that food energy: fat. In addition, over the past 20-years we have also brought into our food supply high fructose corn syrup – which is very unique. High fructose corn syrup is 45 percent fructose and 55 percent glucose and fructose does not require insulin to get within a cell. And at the level of the gylcolysis pathway, the enzyme that gets inhibited is phosphofructokinase, so glycolosis itself gets inhibited at the level of Fructose 6-phosphate. So if you continue to pop large amounts of fructose into the interior of the cell when glycogen stores are full and insulin levels are high you're already shunting towards fat storage, but you're now stacking up high levels of fructose which are very easily synthesized toward triacylglycerol, with the result that you develop a scenario where you not only have high insulin levels to stimulate fat storage, but you also have lots of substrate to work on to create triglycerides for fat storage. So the problem of consuming too many refined carbohydrate, having full glycogen stores and high insulin levels is even more of a problem when you introduce something like high fructose corn syrup because you now have a sugar that can get into the cell regardless of glycogen storage levels and insulin sensitivity. It's like throwing gasoline on the fire of this problem.

CALORIC VALUE OF HIGH-INTENSITY EXERCISE

QUESTION: *I'm curious if you have ever determined what the caloric burn is from a high-intensity workout?*

ANSWER: No form of physical training burns all that many calories. Running a mile, for instance, typically burns (depending upon the subject's bodyweight) roughly 100 calories, so in order to lose a pound of body fat by running you would have to run for 35 miles – and suffer all of the problems inherent with such activities. There have been different sources that have attempted to make similar calculations for calorie burning from high-intensity exercise, but there's a problem in how these are measured. High-intensity exercise creates a situation where, for the exercise to be truly high-intensity in nature, the subject must be within an environment where making such a measurement is difficult to do. Even if there were a means by which one could accurately measure such things, we don't know that knowing those numbers would be all that important because it's not the basis of what we advocate. You should not be dependent upon your exercise sessions as a means of creating a caloric deficit owing to the fact that the human body is far too efficient, and far too evolved for that to work. If we truly believed what the displays on the the treadmills, exercise bikes and ergometers tell us in terms of calorie burn we never would have survived as a species. If we were that calorically inefficient, we would have died hunting and gathering. If we were as calorically inefficient as most treadmills indicate, we would die of starvation while grocery shopping. We need not worry about this as it's not anything we advocate as a reason for exercising. The reason we advocate high-intensity exercise is to enhance our levels of lean muscle mass and to create an overall hormonal metabolic environment that favors lean tissue over body fat.

EPIGENETICS: FOLATE AND FAT LOSS

QUESTION: If folate had such a great effect on turning fat rats into lean rats, why don't we simply add more folate to our diets in order to help us become leaner?

ANSWER: There are probably about 150 genes in which they've found that methylation will change their expression, but it should be remembered that there can be unintended consequences of methylation, which is why we don't advocate supplementing one's diet with folate. And some of these unintended consequences may not manifest for a couple of generations. For instance, a couple of generations back, there was a famine in Scandanavia with the result that now there is a generation in Scandanavia (the descendants of those that lived through the famine) that are presently expressing a higher risk for obesity and diabetes than their forefathers did. So events that have occurred decades ago can have downstream effects for people two generations after the fact that might well be negative.

NAUTILUS NORTH FAT LOSS STUDY

QUESTION: I have heard through the bodybuilding grapevine about a study that John Little did at Nautilus North regarding fat loss and how people who used only two sets once a week (a "Big 2" as it were) made unbelievable progress. What can you tell me about this intriguing study?

ANSWER: The study involved 35 people who were put through a 10 week program that required them to reduce their daily calorie intake by 100 calories (along the lines of Ellington Darden's Nautilus Diet program) every two weeks, starting at a below maintenance level of calories. The diet was a well-balanced diet and did not include supplements of any kind. The subjects started off with a six exercise workout performed once a week (note: these were men and women that had been training in a high-intensity manner at Nautilus North for over one year and varied in age from 20 to 65). Every two weeks, the subjects' daily calorie intake was reduced by 100 calories. But rather than do what Darden did, which was to salt in an additional two to three exercises every two weeks, these subjects went in the opposite direction; after the first two weeks of the study, the subjects had their exercises reduced from six to four; after the next two weeks, the exercises were reduced from four to three, and during the remaining four weeks, half of the subjects stayed on a three exercise program and the other half had their exercises reduced from three to two. Bod Pod testing revealed that the subjects lost a combination of fat and muscle during weeks one and two; they continued to lose fat and muscle during weeks three and four; they lost fat and held muscle during weeks five and six; and the group that stayed with three exercises lost some more fat and did not lose any muscle during weeks seven through ten. The group that cut their exercises to two lost fat and gained muscle during weeks seven through ten. When the data from the study was examined, the conclusion was that two exercises performed for one set each once a week resulted in greater muscle gain and greater fat loss than a three exercise protocol, a four exercise protocol and a six exercise protocol -- despite the subjects being at their lowest calorie intake of the entire program.

I know that when we did a fat loss study at our facility we had several clients who had to miss their weekly workout and came back two weeks later and were stronger and leaner for having done so. The additional recovery period evidently added to their ability to produce the gains that they had stimulated two weeks previously. It must be remembered that what the body is adapting to on a daily basis is *everything* that's going on in one's life and if one is going to have a certain amount of adaptive energy per unit of time, one has to realize that some of that adaptive energy is going to be claimed in the fat loss process. There is a significant metabolic cost to tapping stored body fat and metabolizing it and doing the necessary nutrient partitioning to make an adaptation for what is perceived by the body as being in a potential starvation environment. So that consumes some of that adaptive energy, which, therefore, means that in terms of strength training and muscle gain, this has to be accounted for and probably ratcheted down accordingly. And this is where a lot of people get into trouble because they think of exercise as something that is *burning* calories and burning fat, so when they're trying to lose weight they almost reflexively will ratchet up their activity levels while dieting. And they end up producing too many stressors for the adaptive capabilities that are available and end up becoming overstressed in such a way that their metabolism slows and their cortisol levels spike. Your body is very reluctant to let go of stored bodyfat under those conditions.

-- Doug McGuff, MD

In reviewing the data from the Study presently, we are compelled to look for reasons as to why so little exercise could produce such marked improvement. Perhaps such little exercise is all that is required -- period. Or it could be that the improved fat loss and muscle gain on the subjects who went to two exercises once a week wasn't related at all to the volume changes that occurred over that span of time. Rather it may have been that the subjects were simply performing an appropriate form of exercise for long enough. In other words, it may have been a case of the subjects simply performing high-intensity exercise of varying and decreasing volume over a long enough span of time for a new metabolic dog trail to finally be beaten down. In order for this to happen one has to allow enough time for a new metabolic shift that favors metabolic tissue to gradually come to the fore. And even though it wasn't a "low carbohydrate" diet, per se, by virtue of the low calories in and of themselves, the lower insulin levels that resulted as a consequence of that lower calorie intake would have been quite low, resulting in the creation of a hormonal metabolic environment in the subjects that may not have existed before. And if the subjects were previously consuming a typical North American diet, then that metabolic shift had probably not occurred even in the face of the high-intensity training they had been doing long term. Another explanation might be that through the manipulations in training volume we were discovering a threshold where the economic calculation for the metabolic cost of muscle was changing, so that at a higher volume the stimulus was there but the cost of that stimulus in terms of stress to the organism, and in terms of cortisol production which could thwart the hormonal environment that we were seeking, had a *negative* effect. That is to say, that while we were bringing a proper stimulus to enhance muscle mass in the subjects, in the face of a caloric deficit the volume of the activity was high enough that their bodies made a metabolic calculation for muscle and concluded that it was too expensive to be produced.

In other words, if the activity level or the volume was going to be that high (6 exercises), enhancing muscle mass at that high of a volume would have had too high of a metabolic cost. Consequently, if the body is going to be mobilizing body fat for energy stores and the subjects are going to be that active at that high level of intensity, the metabolic cost of producing muscle tissue may be too high in that context, and, therefore, resulting in muscle being jettisoned along with the fat tissue. Whereas when we started to pull back the volume there was still enough of a stimulus there for muscle tissue to be synthesized but now the cost of that activity and intensity at that level of caloric deficit was no longer a threat, and, therefore, the organism permitted the muscle to be preserved and added to.

WORKOUT FOR FAT LOSS

QUESTION: I would like to ask Dr. McGuff if, in light of the data from the Nautilus North Fat Loss Study, he would change anything about the Body By Science workout program for people that want to lose body fat as their primary goal?

ANSWER: I think I would keep to the same Body By Science program – at least to start. I think it's very conducive to the proper hormonal environment necessary for fat loss. But the problem is that most people are not going to have access to a BodPod, and therefore will not know their compositional data in the way that John uncovered when he conducted his study. Nevertheless, if fat loss is the goal then the primary focus has to be diet with an eye toward keeping the calorie levels low and comprised of lean meats and carbohydrates that are fruit and vegetable based. It would also be important to keep yourself well hydrated for reasons we elucidated in Body By Science. The workout itself should be viewed merely as something that is in place to create the correct environment for fat loss, and if your diet is good but find that things are not going as well as you want, then I think John's data is suggestive that the first place to look would be to reduce the volume or frequency of your training sessions. And while it may seem counter-intuitive, I think the objective data points towards overtraining becoming an even more sensitive issue when you are in a negative calorie balance.

SELYE'S "ADAPTATION ENERGY"

QUESTION: When reading through Dr. Hans Selye's writings on adaptation energy, he indicates that adaptive energy is not simply caloric energy; i.e., it cannot be simply replaced by consuming calories. And to me this sounds almost mystic, as unless you know of a means by which you can detect and measure and locate "adaptive energy" as being something apart from ATP, I have no idea what he could be referring to. Do you?

ANSWER: Keep in mind that sometimes in science you're dealing with a black box of sorts; i.e., something goes in one side and comes out the other and all that you can understand is that the black box has produced some sort of effect. For instance, we don't yet fully understand gravity and all of its implications, but we know enough not to take a step off a 10-storey ledge. We would agree with Dr. Selye, however, that adaptation energy is not caloric (i.e., heat) energy. A large component of it undoubtedly involves hormonal and metabolic shifts and the adaptations that occur as a result of the application of a stressor to the body. That is to say, that the hormonal environment/milieu determines such things as nutrient partitioning and how energy will be utilized. So the significant stressor of bringing the stimulus has to allow time for all of those things to do their job and return to baseline (the catabolic/anabolic balance that we defined in *Body By Science*) and this is much more than just calories. In addition, one needn't be able to measure or quantify something in order to know that it's finite because one can discern its absence fairly easily; after all, "love" is certainly not quantifiable but when someone decides to withdraw it from you, you can certainly tell when it happened. And it is certainly easy to prove that adaptation energy isn't synonymous with calories – otherwise the recovery period following a workout (which for most trainees is seven days) could be hastened to 24 hours if you consumed 7,000 calories beyond your maintenance need of calories, which clearly is not the case.

PART SIX: ATHLETICS

THE PRICE OF ATHLETIC SUCCESS

QUESTION: My son is out of shape and I think being healthy and fit will make a world of difference to his confidence and self-esteem. I look at a lot of professional athletes and they all train more frequently than what you recommend in Body By Science and all of them look to be in awesome shape. What do you think about enrolling my son in a sport or two to get him on the right track?

ANSWER: While many of us look to athletes as being prime examples of physical fitness, what we are really seeing are individuals who have a genetic predisposition to excel at certain physical activities who, through thousands of hours of practice, have become extraordinarily proficient at certain skill sets that are *only* specific to the sport they happen to excel in. What we're *not* seeing is the long-term damage that such athletic training and competition is doing to the bodies of these same individuals. A survey that was conducted with 15,000 athletes from the University of Alabama's alumni department did just that, however, examining the effect that competing in varsity level athletics had on the health and fitness levels of the athletes who participated in them. The authors of the survey concluded that:

> The price many athletes pay to compete is high. Based on these data, some athletes sacrifice their future quality-of-life for their athletic participation in youth athletics, high school, and collegiate sport. Sports are an important part of American culture, but the long-term risks are rarely considered. Increased risk of disability, obesity, and chronic disease may be what a competitive athlete ... will face. [1]

In younger athletes (aged 5 to 14), who are among the most active athletically, the injury rate is equally as shocking. According to the Children's Hospital Boston (the primary pediatric teaching hospital of Harvard Medical School), of the approximately 30 million children and teens who participate in some form of organized sports each year, 3 million of them (or 10 percent) will be hurt as a result. Indeed, one-third of *all* injuries suffered during childhood are caused by their participation in sports. [2]

According to statistics amassed by the National SAFE KIDS Campaign and the American Academy of Pediatrics (AAP):

1.) Sports and recreational activities contribute to approximately 21 percent of all traumatic brain injuries among American children and adolescents.
2.) More than 775,000 children and adolescents ages 14 and under are treated in hospital emergency rooms for sports-related injuries each year. Most of the injuries occurred as a result of falls, being struck by an object, collisions, and overexertion during unorganized or informal sports activities.
3.) More severe injuries occur during individual sports and recreational activities.
4.) Most organized sports-related injuries (60 percent) occur during practice.
5.) Approximately 20 percent of children and adolescents participating in sports activities are injured each year, and one in four injuries is considered serious.
6.) Sports-related injury severity increases with age.
7.) Overuse injury, which occurs over time from repeated motion, is responsible for nearly half of all sports injuries to middle-and high-school students. Immature bones, insufficient rest after an injury, and poor training or conditioning contribute to overuse injuries among children. We will return to this last point later in this chapter.

In terms of injuries incurred on a per sport basis, unless otherwise indicated, the following represents a sample taken just in the United States in 1998, indicating the number of children (aged 5 to 14) who were injured seriously enough to require hospital emergency room treatment, and the various sports that caused these injuries:

- Basketball – 200,000.
- Baseball– 91,000.
- Softball – 26,000 (incidentally, baseball also had the highest fatality rate among sports for children aged 5 to 14, with three to four children dying from baseball injuries each year)
- Bicycling – 320,000 (in addition, 225 children died in bicycle-related accidents in 1997)
- Football – 159,000.
- Gymnastics – 25,500.
- Ice Hockey – 18,000 (statistics from 2001-2002)
- Ice Skating – 10,600.
- In-line skating and/or rollerblading – 27,200.
- Skateboarding – 27,500.
- Sledding – 8,500.
- Snow skiing – 13,500.
- Snow boarding – 9,000.
- Soccer – 77,500.
- Trampoline – 80,000. [3]

In other words, if you choose athletics as the modality of exercise for your son there's a very big risk involved and he will probably be injured either during training or competition, or, like the varsity athletes cited earlier, he could well end up with an "increased risk of disability, obesity and chronic disease." Granted, athletes do develop great motor skills for the specific athletic event in which they compete, but what that has to do with health, fitness or longevity has never been established. What has been established, however, is that participating in sports will take a toll on your health – with very few exceptions. And this is not to suggest that strength training is without risk either, but statistics have shown that even when performed improperly – i.e., in a conventional fashion in which no attention is paid to reducing the forces involved – the percentage of injury is considerably lower than any of the alternate means employed to become stronger and enhance one's health, fitness and functional ability from adolescence to our senior years. In a study conducted by Bian P. Hamill, various sports that were performed within the United Kingdom and the United States were examined and then evaluated based the amount of injuries incurred per 100 hours of participation by the athletes.[4] He summarized his findings as follows:

Multi-Sport Comparative Injury Rates

Sport   Injuries per 100 participation hours

Sport	Injuries per 100 participation hours
Schoolchild soccer	-- 6.20
UK Rugby	-- 1.92
South African Rugby	-- 0.70
UK basketball	-- 1.03
USA basketball	-- 0.03
USA athletics	-- 0.57
UK athletics	-- 0.26
UK Cross-country	-- 0.37
USA Cross-country	-- 0.00
Fives	-- 0.21
P.E.	-- 0.18
Squash	-- 0.10
USA football	-- 0.10
Badminton	-- 0.05
USA gymnastics	-- 0.044
UK tennis	-- 0.07
USA powerlifting	-- 0.0027
USA tennis	-- 0.001
Rackets	-- 0.03
USA volleyball	-- 0.0013
Weight training	-- 0.0035 (85,733 hrs)
Weightlifting	-- .0017 (168,551hrs) [5]

It considering the above statistics it should be pointed out that these take into account *only* those injuries that required hospital emergency room attention, and do not include injuries that were incurred but did not require hospitalization (such as strains, cuts, bruises, etc.), which might well increase these numbers ten fold. Imagine for a moment what would happen if rather than sports events, the above statistics represented the injury rate from jobs or classes in secondary schools. Would you, for instance, be comfortable sending your child into a class knowing that 10 percent of its students would be hurt to the point of requiring emergency room hospitalization or that their attending such classes would result in an "increased risk of disability, obesity and chronic disease?" One would hope not. Indeed, such a class would most likely be cancelled or at least boycotted until major steps were taken to remedy the situation. Nevertheless, when it comes to enrolling our children (or ourselves) in sports it is believed (obviously falsely) by most that the benefits to be had from engaging in such activities largely outweigh the liabilities. Fortunately, as no such impact forces occur with strength training in the manner that we prescribe, such chances of injury are not present, and the benefit of strength training will be that you will create a bigger "shock absorber" for your child's muscles should he decide to participate in athletics. Obviously we are not naive enough to believe that people will be swayed by the data cited above to the point of not allowing their children to participate in sports. Indeed, sports are great fun to watch and great fun to participate in, and people are simply going to do them and want to do them. But, conceding this, we do believe that it is important for a parent to be fully aware of the inherent risks involved in athletics and to take the preventative steps necessary to protect his or her child as fully as possible from the very real threat of injury that his or her child will face. And the best protection for the athlete is to enter competition *stronger*. And having said this, a child can get stronger – without having to risk his or health in sport in order to accomplish it. How? By engaging in a proper strength training program as outlined in *Body By Science*.

SPORT & HEALTH

QUESTION: But doesn't participation in sports make one healthy?

ANSWER: The reality is that there has never been (nor will there ever be) a link between sport and health, or sport and fitness. Everything from the battering athletes take during competition, to the damage caused by many of their rehearsals or practices for competition (recall from above that "Most organized sports-related injuries ... occur during practice"), to the often baseless and dangerous rituals passed along to them by various generations of coaches, to the influx of corporate dollars to embrace equipment, training programs and nutritional practices that – at best – are ineffective, to ingesting powerful performance-enhancing (and often recovery-enhancing) drugs that play havoc with one's arteries and glandular systems, militates against athletics being either healthy or being the best route to enhancing one's fitness. If you're a participant in athletics it becomes even more important for you to become appropriately physically conditioned than it is for most members of the general public because the muscle you build is going to be your major shock absorber and protection from injury.

SKILL CONDITIONING & PHYSICAL CONDITIONING

QUESTION: Your chapter on athletics in Body By Science was fascinating. I was particularly impressed with the distinction you drew between skill conditioning and physical conditioning. However, I'm appalled that most of the coaches that I speak with (even at the Varsity and Professional levels) know little to nothing about this. How can we get the word out?

ANSWER: That's a good question. We put the word out (at least the printed word) in Body By Science, but the rest of the battle will be with people who have this knowledge to make sure that coaches (at least) are introduced to it. A copy of the book can help (many coaches have contacted us to say how much this information improved the performance of their teams and individual players), as does informed dialogue. Now if you can get a coach to grasp this concept – that there is a difference between skill conditioning and physical conditioning – and if you can get him to understand the need to separate them and to have his athletes perform their physical conditioning in a way that meets the requirements of the human body, then you will be well on the way to really doing all that can be done to help him to prepare an athlete to compete at the highest possible level. The problem, however, is getting many coaches to understand this distinction and to act on it. Indeed, most coaches confuse physical conditioning in two respects; one, they think something about the physical conditioning has to mimic the movement or activity of the sport itself (this can be seen in coaches who have their athletes perform explosive Olympic lifting style movements with free weights in order "to have explosive athletes" or by having, say, a baseball player swinging a weighted bat prior to hitting a baseball, or otherwise having athletes performing some sort of movement that mimics a movement in a particular sport). Most coaches have it in their heads that such activities are desirable when in fact they are not the most efficient way of loading muscles (and therefore stimulating muscles to become stronger) as such movements don't effectively track muscle and joint function, and the performance of such activities will (as a matter of mere neuromuscular course) result in a befuddling of the athlete's skill set. This latter point is crucially important because when an athlete is made to perform a movement that is very similar to what will be done in competition but with resistance -- as opposed to how they would normally perform it (without resistance) in a competition -- the result is that the skill isn't learned in a manner that the athlete will encounter in a game situation. Consequently, the learned skill set (throwing heavy weights, for example) has no inherent applicability to the precise athletic environment that it will be used in.

PHYSICAL CONDITIONING & DISCIPLINARY TREATMENT

QUESTION: Last night our hockey team ran out of gas in the third period. I think it was from having two hard practices wherein we were skated hard during the week leading up to our game. Our coach, however, rather than allowing us some "off" days to recharge our batteries,

accused us of being "out of condition" and has
scheduled a 6:00 a.m. practice tomorrow (the day after
our game) in which we will "skate till we puke" in order to
improve our conditioning. What do you think about this?

ANSWER: We think it's ridiculous. What your team
needs now is more recovery time – not another round of
energy-draining activity. Too many coaches embrace
physically-demanding conditioning exercise for purposes
of disciplinary treatment or *esprit de corps* building, or
some form of militaristic "toughening" treatment. You see
this mistake actually glorified in Hollywood treatments
depicting athletic competition, such as the many *Rocky*
movies, and the hockey movie *Miracle On Ice*. In the
hockey movie the audience is led to believe that the
reason why the American team wins the Olympic gold
medal was *because* their coach used hard physical
training as a means of punishment. Another example of
this misconception being glorified was an HBO television
special on Bear Bryant. In the film, Bryant was coaching
the Texas Aggies, and just ran the players into the
ground during the summer months. And as a result of
this the audience is (once again) led to believe that they
became such a well conditioned football team and so
tough that no other team could beat them. While these
are entertaining films, remember that the industry that
produced them refers to itself as "show business" – not
"show science." Virtually everything in terms of the
positive effects of constant hard training on the "skill" of
the athletes depicted is false. Indeed, the exact opposite
is true. If a team is playing poorly or, in your case, was
noted to have "run out of energy" during the third period
of a hockey game (or, for that matter, the fourth quarter
of a football or basketball game), the last thing in a world
a coach should be considering is "punishing" them with
sprint types of activity in their next practice. It's not going
to do anything for the players except undermine their
recovery even further and demoralize them. Such
instances of employing physical training as a means of
punishment, discipline and building *esprit de corps*,
simply does not pay off in any real sense for any team
anywhere. Yes, it most certainly will develop in players a
fear and respect for their coach, but what outcome that

has in terms of performance has really never been established scientifically. Another thing such an approach does is create a situation whereby the coach's actions have succeeded in completely fatiguing the athlete, with the result that the athlete then heads into his competition not fully recovered and not fully capable and, thus, is placed at a much higher risk for injury. We would hazard to say that a lot more injuries occur on the training field and in the training room than ever occur during competition. And, perhaps more importantly, such a coaching approach only serves to shorten athletic careers, because if you chronically overtrain an athlete and the athlete is not permitted sufficient time to fully recover, he is either going to burn out much, much sooner, or suffer a career-ending injury much, much sooner. And this becomes particularly critical during the athlete's competitive season (as opposed to the off season), when the athlete's physiology has to contend not only with games but with practices as well.

"FRESH" SKILLS AND "TIRED" SKILLS

QUESTION: What is the best way for an athlete to practice his skills?

ANSWER: Skills can be practiced under two different scenarios – brief and long. Long duration skill practice is *not* a good option. If you engage in skill practice for too long you develop two different styles -- a *fresh style*, and a *tired style*. And these two different styles involve different pathways between your nervous system and your muscles that, over time, can come to ruin your skills. Rather than having an automatic, ingrained way of jumping, for instance, an athlete's body will instead have two styles, or pathways, and in the heat of competition, confusion about which pathway to choose will inhibit proper performance of the skill. If, instead, the athlete has paid attention to performing his physical conditioning properly, and he pays attention to full recovery, he should only have to rely on the *fresh style*. The best way to practice skills is using brief sessions that are repeated frequently. Rather than performing two continuous hours of skill training, the athlete is better served by performing 10-minute sessions with 5-minutes of rest in between. If he becomes tired he should perform the drill and then rest for 10-minutes. If he gets get too tired, he should terminate his practice and, if possible, come back later in the day (or the next day) to resume it. It is much better to put in 15-minutes of skill training every day than it is to put in 2 hours once a week. This pattern of practice avoids the *fresh-tired* confusion issue and also allows for *repetition*; that is to say, repetition of a skill in a non-fatigued state (i.e., exactly as it is performed in competition). This is the key to improvement. In general, we recommend that the athlete limit his skill set training to only one or two skills per practice. It must be remembered, however, that specific sports skills are always incorporated in a broad focus environment. We therefore recommend linking the skill with a scrimmage or at least performing it at top speed (as it would be in a game). If an athlete constantly practices his skills at half speed, then he will develop the skill *only* at *that* speed. By contrast, if he practices the skill at full speed, such as he would in an all-out competition (such as during a shift in a hockey game or running for a pass in football game), the athlete will then develop the ability to execute that skill at top speed. So, we would recommend that an athlete practice his or her skills in brief but frequent sessions, and be sure to tie it all together with a game-situation scrimmage during each practice session.

A RECOMMENDED PHYSICAL TRAINING FREQUENCY

QUESTION: How often should an athlete strength train?

ANSWER: In terms of physical training (rather than skill training, which can be done daily) for athletes, the best way to proceed would be to workout once a week during the off season and then, depending upon how hectic the competitive season is, the workouts should be cut back to perhaps once every two weeks. The reason for the reduced frequency of physical training workouts during the competitive season is because of the toll that the practices (particularly the way practices are currently performed as a mix of skill and conditioning training) and competition takes. The once a week physical conditioning workouts should also be spaced such that they are distanced from the athlete's skill conditioning in order that the fatigue-related component of the skill conditioning activity doesn't compromise the strength training component. Spacing them out this way will also preclude the strength training workouts from interfering with the athlete's skill conditioning practice, meaning that the athlete has to have some reasonable degree of recovery take place before he or she starts working on their skill sets, so as not to confuse the skill sets. And then, during the competitive season, the workouts should be pulled back to once every 14-days, as the demands of the season are going to be considerable. The athlete (and/or coach) can then adjust from there depending upon how things appear to be going on the athlete's progress chart/workout record. During the season the athlete should at least be maintaining his strength or progressing it. If the athlete witnesses any retrogression of his strength, then he should either throttle back a little bit on the intensity of his workouts or allow even more time to elapse before his next workout to allow for a full recovery to take place.

THE RISK OF STRETCHING

QUESTION: I was fascinated in Body By Science to read that the scientific literature does not favor stretching before a competition. None of my athlete buddies (who all stretch before engaging in their sports activities) believe it. Can you tell me anything more about the downside of stretching for athletes?

ANSWER: Certainly If you were you to look at an electron microscopic study of a muscle at rest you will note that there is a partial overlapping of the heads of the actin and myosin filaments such that if the myosin heads were to engage you would produce maximal force generation from that position. But if you overstretch a muscle and separate the "Z-bands" farther apart you set up a situation such that when the myosin heads engage with the actin filaments (such as they would if an athlete were to produce a forceful muscular contraction, as in sprinting) they will be doing so from a position of very poor mechanical leverage, which will dramatically raise the odds of their being subject to tears and separations at the microscopic level (and, therefore, at the macroscopic level). If one were able to achieve any lengthening at the sarcomere level, it would only be accomplished to the detriment of the athlete owing to the increased risk for tears and injury. Stretching before an athletic event is worse than simply being the wrong thing to do, owing to the fact that it's not even in a ballpark where it can be assessed as "wrong." It's simply a non-rational activity. And this not to suggest that stretching is always a bad thing. We know, for example, that stretching, per se, during certain phases of rehabilitation (which is done for a deranged or injured joint) can actually have some therapeutic benefit. For instance, if someone has had a ligamentous disruption in his knee and has a blood effusion in his knee, a physical therapist who provides gentle stretching force in both flexion and extension can help to keep the knee joint mobile during the period of time when it's healing (and this actually serves some purpose). But the fact that this activity is of some benefit to an injured athlete does not translate to it being of any benefit to an uninjured athlete (or even a team of them).

STRETCHING AND COACHING RITUALISM

QUESTION: So why has stretching been so ingrained in our coaching psyches?

ANSWER: One answer is that it is complementary to the ritualism inherent in sports. It's something that can be done in a group setting, which reinforces *esprit de corps* and has a certain mystical component to it because it's something that a team can do in unison. This is the same reason, in fact, that the military teaches soldiers to march in units; i.e., it produces this feeling of solidarity. And when such activity is performed before a competition it psychologically announces to everyone involved that, "We are getting ready for competition" in much the same way that Russell Crowe's character in the movie "Gladiator" always picked up a handful of dirt out of the gladiatorial arena and rubbed it into his palms prior to engaging in battle. It is done largely for the same reason that virtually every sports team (particularly in the United States) gathers around in a circle for a team "prayer" prior to a game. Now leaving aside the implications of this for a minute, stretching before a game is largely done for the same reason; i.e., it's simply a quasi-religious mystical rite that announces to all that you're preparing for competition. And this is not to suggest that there is anything wrong with pre-game rituals that announce to yourself and others that you are getting ready for competition, but the truth is that what you choose to be your team ritual could be anything; i.e., it could be an inspirational song (a team song) that allows a minute or two for the team to become settled and focused and quiet as they listen to it in the locker room before the game. This would (and does) help a player and his teammates to get psyched up and prepared. The problem with stretching is that it is an activity that (unlike the prayer or the team song) can actually cause harm to your athletes.

FOOTBALL PLAYERS AND OXYGEN MASKS

QUESTION: What is the reason that some football players strap on an oxygen mask when they come off the field?

ANSWER: We don't think there is any reason for this. The first problem with such a procedure is that the partial pressure of oxygen in the ambient air is more than adequate to saturate a player's hemoglobin molecules 100 percent with oxygen. Indeed, that's how oxygen is transported to his tissues; i.e., hemoglobin comes in through the lungs and the blood flow through the lungs picks up the oxygen. It then becomes saturated with it, and carries it to the working muscles and the organs so that oxygen is delivered to the tissues at that level. And, at room air, a player is going to be receiving as much oxygen on his hemoglobin as his hemoglobin can hold.

By supplying additional oxygen his hemoglobin oxygen saturation will *not* be increased one iota. Such a practice actually is the reverse of what most athletes should be doing, which is blowing off carbon dioxide. Once an athlete has produced a lactic acidosis his blood pH drops, and the way you quickly correct a blood pH drop is to hyperventilate and blow off carbon dioxide. If you don't do this, the dissolved carbon dioxide in the blood will produce carboxylic acid and worsen the acidosis. And an athlete's ability to blow off carbon dioxide determines just how quickly he can correct that acidosis. And should he then put on an oxygen mask thinking that he needs more oxygen (which he's already 100 percent saturated with), the mask will actually trap the carbon dioxide that he should be trying to blow off and he re-breathes it. Thus, by putting an oxygen mask over his face he is actually prolonging the process of recovering from exertion, rather than improving it. Most athletes would do almost as well to hold a pillow over their face.

THE POST-GAME STATIONARY BIKE

QUESTION: *I always see hockey players being interviewed after a game while riding a stationary bike. I asked my coach about this and he said they were doing it to "get rid of lactic acid" in their legs, which helps them recover. Is this true?*

ANSWER: No it's not. The way lactic acid is metabolized out of the body is by being circulated through the body via a process involving the venous return, which takes it through the central vein of the liver. Once in the liver a metabolic cycle called the Cori Cycle converts the excess lactate into pyruvate and then reverse engineers it through the glycolysis cycle to create glucose through a process known as gluconeogenesis. This process takes the lactate that accumulates in a well-conditioned athlete's muscles and uses it as nitrous so that it can be recycled back to glucose by the athlete for reuse. And this is exactly what happens during the recovery period when the athlete is no longer exerting himself. The use of a stationary bike is only helpful if one is attempting to deflate a "pump" in the legs, whereby light cycling can create a condition where the venous congestion or the "pump" in the legs can be resolved a little bit quicker. What happens during high levels of muscular exertion, such as racing hard on a bicycle, is that the cyclist will produce a high level of arterial blood flow into the working muscles and as the working muscles are contracting and, depending upon the position of the legs while the athlete is cycling, some venous blood can be trapped in the extremity that's being worked and produce a feeling of congestion or pump. In such cases, mild post event cycling can work if they're set up in the correct position; i.e., where the legs are not flexed too acutely, the seat of the stationary bicycle is high and the legs are able to fully extend. This will produce just enough muscle contraction to milk the venous blood out of the area but not produce enough arterial demand for more blood to be delivered into the extremities. So, in the case of cyclists at least, they are, to some extent, decompressing some of the venous compression in their legs, which might make their legs *feel* better – but this has nothing to do with flushing out lactic acid. And, as it relates to hockey players after a game – if getting rid of lactic acid is the goal -- what works just as well for this purpose is just simply standing and/or walking around a little bit after the game has ended. Just the activity of doing this will diminish the congestion in the legs equally as effectively. There's nothing magical about getting on a stationary bike, perhaps other than it makes you look special. In hockey, when the game is over, each member of the team usually skates down to congratulate their goalie, then they skate over to the bench to exit the ice, and then they walk down a corridor to the change room, walk into the change room and then – finally – sit down and remove their equipment. And by then the lactic acid is pretty well gone from their legs anyway. Sitting on a stationary bike at this point does nothing. To get rid of congestion in the legs, however, all you have to do is have a situation where your legs are relatively straight and you're doing some light contraction with the legs. That allows the congested venous blood to return from the legs. By standing or walking you will place the joint angles where they're not acute and thus not impinging any blood flow out of the lower extremities.

This will allow the congestion or "pump" in the legs to resolve a little bit more quickly.

WEIGHTED BATS

QUESTION: I'm wondering what your opinion is on baseball players swinging a weighted bat? Every time before a batter goes to the plate, he steps into the batter's box. En route he puts a weighted "donut" on his bat and then takes several practice swings with it. What is the thinking behind this?

ANSWER: The thinking is, "Well, if I swing a heavier bat right before I get up to bat, then a regular bat is going to feel lighter and I'm going to hit the ball harder." When in fact what he's doing is neurologically befuddling that particular skill set immediately before he goes to perform it. He really couldn't choose a worse thing to do than to swing a weighted bat. But this activity has, like stretching and oxygen masks, become a sort of ritual that's ingrained into the game. And the people that are able to hit home runs after doing this are simply getting home runs *in spite* of doing this rather than *because* of doing this. It's another example of the "tall trees in the canopy" analogy in that there are people that have nervous systems that are able to discriminate very finely; i.e., they have a fine tune button on their skill sets and they can discriminate one skill set from another very easily. Most people, however, cannot do this. And it just so happens that outstanding athletes that display outstanding skills also tend to have an outstanding type of nervous system that makes them good discriminators in this regard. As a result, if the vast majority of the population attempted to engage in such an activity it would only serve to befuddle and mess up that skill set for them. But for the athlete with the ability to discriminate skill sets at a high level, he can engage in such activities will no ill effect because he possesses the genetic ability to be able to discriminate the two different skill sets even when they are very similar in nature. You'll also note that those athletes that are good discriminators are also athletes that can excel at multiple sports. Deon Sanders, for instance, can play an NFL football game and a Major League Baseball game on the same day – and do well in both games because he is a good neuromuscular discriminator. There just are certain people, neurologically, that have this ability to make such high level distinctions with regard to skill sets. Unfortunately it would appear that it's the best athletes that can do it and get away with it, and consequently their genetic endowment in this regard serves to perpetuate the myth that doing such activities will work for the majority of athletes who aren't able to make these subtle neurological discriminations (and for whom it actually makes matters worse).

CROSS TRAINING DEBUNKED

QUESTION: In Body By Science *you relate how the concept of "Cross Training" is without scientific base. I'm still not clear on how becoming proficient in more sports than less sports can hurt an athlete's performance in his own sport. Can you explain this to me?*

ANSWER: Remember that the learning of sports-specific skills are *very* specific and they do *not* transfer to other sports. In his book *The New Bodybuilding for Old-School Results* (available online at: www.drdarden.com) Ellington Darden revealed what might have been the closest thing we've yet seen to the actual results of "cross-training" in action. Darden recalled a television series that was broadcast in the late 1970s called the "Superstars" competition. In this competition, superstars from various sporting disciplines, such as Johnny Bench from baseball, Johnny Unitas from football, Jean Claude Killy from skiing, Joe Frazier from professional boxing, Elvin Hayes from baseball, Emerson Fittipaldi from car racing and Bob Seagren from the discipline of pole vaulting, came to Rotunda, Florida to compete in ten sporting events that were different from their particular specialty. These athletes competed in such things as bowling, rowing, swimming, cycling golf, tennis and weightlifting. Surprisingly to many people, these athletes who were so outstanding in their particular sport were embarrassingly bad in the other athletic activities; Joe Frazier was next to useless in the swimming pool, and despite being a one time heavyweight boxing champion of the world, struggled to press a modestly weighted barbell overhead; Johnny Unitas had trouble rowing his boat, and Hayes couldn't hit a tennis ball properly. Anyone who witnessed the Dave Mirra tour on ESPN may recall Dave trying to learn wakeboarding. If skill was a generalized thing, he should have been pulling spins and flips on the first run. Instead, he spent the day getting a lake water enema. The reason, again, being that skill training for a particular sport develops skills particular to that sport -- period. And these skills are not transferable to other sports (and sometimes this also applies to different positions within a particular sport, such as the skills necessary to become a good defenseman, forward or goalie in hockey). The *Superstars* athletes had never practiced or developed the skills that were specific to the sporting activities they were made to participate in during this competition. This was before the prize money for these contests increased to the point where the athletes who competed actually began to practice the specific sports activities that they would be performing in the competition. Remember: Practice makes perfect, but only when perfectly practiced.

OVERTRAINING SKILLS

QUESTION: Given that you can overtrain in terms of physical conditioning, is it also possible that you can likewise overtrain a skill set?

ANSWER: Absolutely. An interesting aside to skill training is that it is possible to develop a skill to such a high level that the brain will no longer discriminate that particular skill at all. This results in a sudden seizure of skill such that you can no longer perform it anymore. This phenomenon has been noted particularly in concert pianists and professional violinists and string players who perform thousands of movements per day. The condition is called Focal Hand Dystonia – and here is how it comes into play: On the motor strip of the brain each individual finger has a separate representation, but musicians can become so skilled in their ability to perform rapid movements with their fingers that the neurological impulses can no longer keep up and the individual finger representation on the motor strip gets blurred. In other words, their finger movements are now occurring so rapidly that they summate and overlap, and the five separate fingers now become represented as one individual unit on the motor strip. And when the musician who develops this condition attempts to produce any rapid finger movement, rather than just the one finger he's wanting to activate, the brain consolidates every playing action onto one location of the motor strip with the result that all five (or ten) of his fingers will spasmodically activate, rather than rapid isolated finger movement. It used to be thought that this was some sort of psychological problem or a rebellion against the discipline it took to be a musician at that level, but what science has found is that it is actually a neurological disorder that is a by-product of becoming too proficient at a particular skill level. It's a form of neurological overtraining that causes this to happen and evidently the only way to get around it is to start, very laboriously, working each individual finger over again very slowly so that one can recreate the individuation and representation of each digit on the motor strip of the brain again -- and then build up from there. So skill training can actually become so proficient that it produces focal dystonia, which might also be an indicator that one can overtrain skill practice just as one might overtrain physical conditioning and that, at extremely high levels of development, one might be running the risk of hindering one's dexterity with excessive skill practice, rather than enhancing it.

TRAINING FREQUENCY
FOR ATHLETES

QUESTION: How frequently should an athlete workout during the off-season and then during the competitive season to build or maintain his strength?

ANSWER: The workouts we advocate for athletes in *Body By Science* should be performed no more than once every seven days on an alternating basis during the off-season. During the competitive season, the frequency of these workouts may have to be spaced out to once every two weeks. And do not add any exercises into these programs, as they should never exceed five (at most) per workout in order to ensure that the athlete is giving 100 percent to each exercise, each and every workout.

PRE-SEASON METABOLIC CONDITIONING

QUESTION: How soon before the season should an athlete begin his metabolic conditioning training?

QUESTION: The metabolic conditioning that is lost after a season ends can be recovered quite quickly, often times in as little as two weeks prior to the start of the next season. However, the strength conditioning that is required should be allowed a little more time, typically up to two months leading up to the season for most athletes. The reason for this time discrepancy is that metabolic adaptations can ramp up very quickly; i.e., you can stimulate and produce specific metabolic adaptations in most players in the two or three weeks leading up to the competitive season. And then you can rely – if the season is busy enough – entirely on the competition to maintain the appropriate metabolic conditioning. Strength training, however, requires longer as you're asking your athletes' bodies to make a considerably greater metabolic investment in the creation of new tissue.

TABATA PROTOCOL

QUESTION: How often could the Tabata protocol be performed for metabolic conditioning in preparation for the competitive season?

ANSWER: The Tabata Protocol is very demanding, and uses up resources that could otherwise be employed for full recovery of the athlete. So the athlete would want to be very careful with this because if he performed the

Tabata Protocol during the off-season for conditioning along with strength training, he'd still be seven days recovering from the strength workout and then perhaps another seven days would be required to recover from the Tabata workout. The best way to keep this in mind is to always make sure that you understand (and, without fail, almost every athlete we've ever worked with or any coach that we've ever encountered, has never even considered the concept) that *competition is training*. And not only is competition training, it is the *ultimate* training. It is the ideal workout for mimicking the metabolic conditioning that one needs for a specific sport, and it's the ideal workout for working on the skill set that one requires for one's specific sport. And, as with all training, it takes a toll on one's recovery ability that needs to be accounted for. So competition is training and it may be that during the season, in terms of metabolic conditioning, if the athlete's schedule is busy enough, competition may be all that any athlete needs.

NOT THAT DIFFERENT

QUESTION: In Body By Science *a lot of the training programs for individual sports seem similar. Doesn't a football player require the strengthening of different muscles than a hockey player?*

ANSWER: What many athletes are sensing as they read the workouts recommended for their particular sport in *Body By Science* is that there is a commonality to them, and they feel a little bit underwhelmed that the needs of their specific sport aren't considered that much more special than the needs of athletes in any other sport. But in reality the musculature needs to be addressed almost identically in any athlete because all athletes should want to be as strong as possible throughout their entire body – and we all have the *same* muscle groups in our bodies, whether we're basketball players or golfers. And a simple approach such as we've prescribed is always best because it leaves the athlete's recovery ability relatively undisturbed, which allows plenty of time and energy for specific skill training -- which is where the athlete must spend the bulk of his training time to excel in his or her particular sport.

SKILL TRAINING AFTER CONDITIONING TRAINING

QUESTION: *How soon after a workout can an athlete perform his skill training?*

ANSWER: If an athlete performs a workout along the lines of what we advocate in *Body By Science*, he or she should be able to perform his or her skill training within two days. The day after the strength training workout, however, would be better spent relaxing and reviewing competitive data, such as watching video of the last game or competitive event. The day after a competition, while the events of the game are still fresh in the athlete's mind, is an ideal time to be reviewing game film and performing mental practice.

MENTAL PRACTICE

QUESTION: *What kind of "mental practice" are you referring to?*

ANSWER: Any sort of meditative protocol whereby you mentally practice enhancing skill sets has been shown to be essentially as effective as the skill practice itself. And when you combine skill practice and mental practice together they have an enhanced effect on improving athletic performance.

PLANNING A TRAINING SCHEDULE

QUESTION: *I am a coach of a football team and I don't want my athletes overtrained and possibly injured. But the season's schedule makes this impossible. Wouldn't you agree that most sports have too hectic a schedule and, given this, what should a coach do to prevent overtraining?*

ANSWER: When we strength train the general public we

know by simply looking at a client's workout chart if he or she has recovered sufficiently. A quick glance at a progress chart reveals how much weight a trainee is using, his current Time Under Load, how many repetitions he performed with a given weight, and the time it took him to complete his workout. However, this process becomes a little trickier with regard to athletic recovery (unless you can employ high-tech body composition testing, which can be expensive) but the bottom line, again, is performance. Most coaches are able to tell when an athlete is flat and when he is not. It's interesting to note that some of the most astounding performances occur in athletes that are coming off of an injury. And the reason for this is that an injury often forces them *not to train at all* prior to the competition. In other words, for the first time in months the athlete has been given "off time" which allowed his system to fully recover. For example, the UCI World Championships in BMX were won by athletes that had been out of competition for a period of three months or more. Indeed, the 2000/2001 World Cup was won by a rider that had broken his thumb at the very beginning of the season -- he had a complex fracture that required a prolonged recovery period -- but he won the World Championships because all of the other riders were still on the competitive circuit and almost burned out by the time the World Competition rolled around. By contrast, he had been off recuperating from his injury, so he was able to come into this competition with fresher legs than anyone else had and he tore through the competition. In sports such as BMX, every year brings forth a new rider that just turned pro who comes up quick and for one or two years will completely dominate and look like he's going to be a new phenom in the sport. But invariably within 18 to 24-months he's a mid-pack rider because the competitive circuit in BMX is too thick with competitions at the professional level. Just by virtue of the racing schedule alone, the athletes are chronically overtrained. To make matters worse, most of them are very competitive and compulsive and try to engage in physical training and skill training in the weeks in between competitions. As a result, chronic overtraining develops and they become flat. And when an amateur comes up into the ranks he comes in fresh without a chronically overtrained body and that freshness allows him to dominate for about the first 12 to 18 months until he, too, accumulates enough chronic wear, tear and overtraining and falls back into the middle of the pack with the rest of them. And this is a snapshot in miniature of just about every competitive sport – from minor to professional sports. In the NHL, they play eighty-plus games in a season, and then have weekly practices and then playoff quarter finals, semi finals and the Stanley Cup championship (plus an all-star game thrown into the mix), so the players end up overtrained, with many hockey players becoming injured throughout the season. It is not a coincidence that during the 2007-2008 season the Tampa Bay Lightning NHL team had the fewest injuries of any professional hockey team and they also held *fewer* practices in between games than any other NHL team. It would be optimal for athletes if they could scale back the volume of their competitions or games to allow them to be healthier and better able to perform at their highest levels. This would also reduce the chances of overtrained-induced sluggishness and potentially career-ending injuries. The problem is – and this is the "norm" in virtually every sport, particularly if you have an exceptional athlete – is that sport is an animal that eats its young. If you're an exceptional performer, let's say a running back who gets drafted to the NFL, the team will over utilize that athlete to the point where they just grind him into the ground. A lot of NFL teams would be better served to conduct their draft around their talented athletes in such a way that they not overplay them.

GENETICS AND ATHLETIC SUCCESS

QUESTION: *I know that genetics are crucially important in terms of muscle building potential. What is its relationship to athletic success?*

ANSWER: While both physical training and skill training are important to you as an athlete, from a more aerial view of the whole process it needs to be understood that the genetic factor is huge in determining athletic success and dominance. You can become a good athlete through proper skill conditioning and physical conditioning, but to become a truly great athlete, truly world class, requires proper skill and physical conditioning -- and genetics. And when it comes to high level competitive sports – collegiate football, professional football, hockey, baseball, soccer, golf, etc. – a lot of this ridiculous folklore that we've been discussing has come out of the coaching world because they have given to them athletes that have emerged through a vicious natural selection process. These are the type of genetically gifted individuals that one could train in almost any fashion and they would still show outstanding results. Unfortunately, most people do *not* share in the same genetic gifts of the elite athlete. As a consequence, poor training practices that are better tolerated by the genetically gifted athlete reinforce a lot of very primitive superstitious coaching folklore. But if one really steps back and rationally analyzes the situation of every dynamic winning team, you will note, as we do in *Body By Science*, that winning teams are produced by scouts, not by coaches. Talent scouting is the thing that makes an outstanding team. If you can skim the cream of the genetic crop to build your team, then the odds are that you will have a winning team. And if ideal genetics are combined with a scientifically sound training program such as indicated in *Body By Science*, athletic success is sure to follow.

PART SEVEN: SAFETY

STRENGTH TRAINING: BENEFIT VS. RISK

QUESTION: I love the benefits of strength training that you listed in Body By Science. *However, you mentioned in the book that exercise can be likened to medicine, and that the stronger the effect of a particular medicine, the stronger the potential side effects. Does this mean that because the benefits are greatest with strength training that the risks are also greatest?*

ANSWER: The medical literature is full of studies that reveal the many benefits of strength training. These studies have revealed that strength training improves one's mood, improves insulin sensitivity, improves blood lipid profiles, produces less risk of falls in the elderly, and decreased risk of colon cancer. In addition, strength training has not only been shown to be a great means of enhancing cardiovascular efficiency, but is also the safest means of achieving this goal. What is important to keep in mind is that the muscles truly are the windows to your body. They are the mechanism by which we can stress and stimulate all of the body's support systems (cardiovascular, respiratory, skeletal, metabolic, endocrine, etc.) and the higher the quality of the muscular work in your exercises, the greater the positive effect you will have on all of your body's systems. Your question is an excellent one, as all of the foregoing notwithstanding this is not to say that there is "zero" risk and only upside with this activity, nor to say that proper resistance training is ideal for all people. Nevertheless, it remains an almost perfect activity for its ability to produce substantial benefits in minimum time and for its relative safety as compared to other popular forms of physical activity.

KEEPING THE FORCES LOW

QUESTION: What's the big deal with lower forces in exercise? You seem to make a big point of it in Body By Science.

ANSWER: The reason that we advocate a slow, smooth cadence of muscular contraction and a selection of weights that produces a sequential recruitment of motor units is that doing so limits the amount of force that one encounters when one exercises. The really interesting thing about high-intensity training is that the higher the intensity gets during a given set of exercise, and the more rapidly you are weakening and fatiguing yourself, the safer the workout becomes. In all other forms of exercise – from dance aerobics to jogging – anything you do in an attempt to try to raise the intensity results in disproportionately raising the forces your body is subjected to. Consequently, if you go from jogging to sprinting, or from low impact to high impact aerobics, the forces will rise exponentially. And the problem with these approaches is that the consequences of performing them typically do not occur acutely. The consequences of these force issues come home to roost 15 to 20-years later. And that's why so much bad exercise has been successfully promulgated upon the public: because the ugly consequences of such exercises don't really rear their heads until 20-years later when your hips and knees are arthritic. And one of the many things that proper resistance exercise affords you is a means of enhancing the stimulus/intensity but doing so in a way that protects you from excessive forces that are going to have long-term negative consequences.

WARMING UP

QUESTION: *What do you recommend for a warm up prior to exercising with the "Big 5" routine?*

ANSWER: A regimented warm up is not necessary with the type of workout program that we advocate. While a warm up is important for sporting activities that involve high forces (through impact) and that involve the tandem recruiting of motor units that are going to produce high force, such force factors are not present with proper exercise. With the type of exercise that we advocate the warm-up is built in as motor units are sequentially recruited and fatigued. The first repetitions of each set actually serve as the warm up for the higher levels of exertion to follow, and by the time one reaches the final repetitions of a set (the ones involving the highest levels of exertion) one has fatigued to the point where one is now too weak to hurt oneself.

PROPER BREATHING

QUESTION: I've been told by a personal trainer that you must "breathe in while you are lowering the weight and breathe out while lifting the weight." Is this good advice?

ANSWER: This is bad advice on a number of fronts. First, it is needlessly complex and difficult to coordinate. Second, as the demands of the work become more severe (that is, as you fatigue and the intensity grows higher), you are going to be producing more lactic acid, and this will serve to drive a higher respiratory rate. Consequently, if you try to peg your breathing rate to the cadence of the work you're doing, as your respiratory rate increases you may end up increasing the speed of your repetitions to keep pace. This is unwise, as a quicker repetition pace can open the door to increased momentum and amplified force issues that can lead to injury. A wiser path to take with regard to breathing is simply to keep your mouth open during the exercise and breathe freely, which will break any association between synchronizing Val Salva to high levels of muscular output. This is somewhat counter-intuitive, in the sense that typically any time one is under strain to try to lift a heavy object they will automatically Val Salva for the simple reason that by trapping venous blood in a working muscle, one can actually engorge the muscle and increase the force dissipated from the soft tissue itself, thus providing an internal mechanical assist whenever one holds one's breath. However, doing so will short circuit the inroading process (which is the goal of proper training) and, by synchronizing breath holding with a high level of force output, one can produce a dangerous increase in blood pressure. When you have the urge to hold your breath during a set, *that* is the time to actually breath faster in a form of hyperventilation. When we notice that a client is starting to slow down to the point where moving the resistance is becoming very difficult for them, we instruct them to breathe like they're trying to blow the weight up. It is important that one's breathing be what it needs to be relative to the level of one's exertion and fatigue, because as one develops more lactic acidosis one's respiratory rate naturally rises. Consequently, if a trainee has the urge to hold his breath he should break that urge by deliberately breathing faster. Doing so actually prevents him from synchronizing a Val Salva with high levels of exertion, which is a scenario whereby one can produce spikes in blood pressure that compromise venous return, which can then lead to a sudden drop in cardiac output, making one more prone to fainting.

GRIPPING TIGHTLY

QUESTION: Is it a good idea to avoid gripping the handles on exercise machines too tightly while exercising?

ANSWER: Yes. Tight gripping, particularly done in conjunction with Val Salva, can create a scenario whereby one traps venous blood in a particular area of the body, such as in the extremity being trained. And, again, if this is performed in conjunction with Val Salva, one will increase the intra thoracic pressure in such a way that it is greater than the venous return pressure to the heart, thus slowing the flow of venous return to the heart. And as the venous return to the heart is what determines the cardiac output ejected from the left ventricle, the backwash of blood that occurs during diastole is what determines one's coronary artery blood flow. So not only does one unnecessarily raise blood pressure with tight gripping and Val Salva, but one also decreases the volume of return of venous blood to the right side of the heart which therefore affects the amount of blood ejected out of the left side of the heart, which, in turn, effects the amount that backwashes into the coronary arteries. So by gripping too tightly and holding one's breath one can create a situation whereby blood pressure is higher (which means that one is now having to push against greater resistance), but cardiac return (and therefore coronary artery blood flow) is being compromised, and that is a situation that is undesirable and potentially dangerous.

GRIPPING ON PULLDOWNS AND ROWS

QUESTION: If gripping tightly can raise an individual's blood pressure, what, then, can one do on exercises where gripping tightly is unavoidable, such as the Pulldown or Compound Row?

ANSWER: We don't worry about gripping with these exercises too much because, in this context, the gripping is occurring in conjunction with movement of the extremity where the gripping is involved. Where gripping really becomes a problem is during certain isometric movements and particularly when it's coordinated with a Val Salva maneuver. What we wish to teach our readers, and what we teach our clients, is a continuous breathing method that does not allow any breath holding or Val Salva whatsoever. The real marked rises in blood pressure occur when you hold your breath and push against a closed glottis or do the Val Salva maneuver. That, in conjunction with forceful gripping, will raise one's blood pressure to a high level, but it's really not known if that is acutely dangerous or not because the elevated blood pressure that's being measured may not necessarily be intervascular pressure but rather the compartmental pressures of the muscles and connective tissues that result from gripping. The forceful gripping that's necessary in a pulling movement we don't believe to be dangerous, if it's done in a context of actually moving the limb that is attached to that gripping element, because then you're getting venous return through that limb and you're not coordinating it with any Val Salva maneuver.

ANYEURYSM & EXERCISE

QUESTION: I've heard of people suffering a stroke or anyeurysm during exercise. And two of the exercises that I've heard about this occurring on were Overhead

Pulldowns and Overhead Presses. Any comments?

ANSWER: Anyeurysms are largely genetic in nature, with the result that the people you mentioned could have suffered an aneurysms simply while driving to their gyms. If you have that sort of a genetic predisposition to aneurysm, then exerting yourself and performing a Val Salva maneuver can definitely lead to problems. And it's important that the reader keep in mind that while exercise (and strength training in particular) can provide tremendous health and fitness benefits to people, it is not a "risk-free" activity, and those sort of unforeseen things can strike you. But by the same token, those sort of straws that break the camel's back can occur in all sorts of day-to-day activities; i.e., when you're straining to pick up something heavy or straining during a bowel movement – all of those things produce similar concomitant rises in blood pressure. So life is not a risk-free event and the death rate is the same for everyone -- one per customer – which makes a lower force approach to exercise even more important when considering what type of fitness program one should employ.

EXERCISE-INDUCED HEADACHE

QUESTION: I've heard of a condition called "Exercise-Induced Headache." What do you know about this?

ANSWER: Ironically, Exercise-Induced Headache (EIH) is a side effect that can occur as a result of a desirable effect that appropriate strength training can produce; namely, the milking of venous blood out of the veins back to the heart as a result of intensely contracting muscles massaging the veins in the working extremities. However, sometimes this venous return can exceed the compliance capability of the heart, and one can produce an enhanced venous blood pressure toward the cerebral circulation that stretches the cerebral dural sinuses in the brain. And this is what triggers an EIH. It's important to know that EIH, while extremely unpleasant, is nonetheless harmless and is a condition that seems to particularly strike those who are badly deconditioned (more so than those who are least modestly fit). Since a lot of what damps venous blood flow to the brain is the tonus of the upper body musculature, it is a condition that tends to occur when one's upper body musculature has become atrophied over time. It can also occur as a result of excessive holding of breath and Val Salva that can occur during exercise. Thus, by not holding one's breath during exercise one can go a long way toward preventing such occurrences. Another factor that can help to prevent this condition from occurring has to do with the sequence in which one performs one's exercises; i.e., if the larger muscle exercises (such as the leg press) that produce a lot of cephalic venous blood flow are performed towards the end of the workout, the exercises that one performs prior to this will serve to create a pump in the upper body musculature that will then damp some of the venous blood flow. Another way to avoid EIH is to perform neck exercises (i.e., neck flexion and neck extension) at the beginning of one's workout. This will serve to cause the neck musculature to have an even more profound pump and, thus, damp the venous blood flow towards the head. Again, in terms of safety considerations, an EIH is not really a dangerous event but it is a very unpleasant event that one should seek to avoid. It is an event that is more likely to occur in beginners to strength training and, surprisingly, is more common in female subjects, particularly middle aged females, because they tend to have preservation of lower extremity muscle mass and atrophy of their upper extremity muscle mass. As a result, when performing a Leg Press or large muscle movement, they're still able to produce a significant northward flow of venous blood but in the context of an atrophied upper body that can't damp that blood flow towards the brain. If an EIH starts to manifest, the best remedy is to terminate the workout right then and there -- it's over for that day. It's also important to explain to a client that if it happens to them that it's okay to shut the workout down and quit for the day because any attempt to try and "work through it" will only result in the condition markedly worsening and then persisting for several days afterwards before it settles down.

LIGHT HEADEDNESS AND NAUSEA

QUESTION: I've just started high-intensity training and during my workouts I feel a little light-headed and nauseous. Is this common?

ANSWER: It is not unheard of for trainees to occasionally experience feelings of light-headedness or nausea during or immediately after a high-intensity workout. This is not something to fear, but it is something that can and should be avoided with a clear understanding of the process that triggers it. The nausea that one feels is a result of burning so much glycogen out of the muscles that the body attempts to continue muscular contraction by manufacturing more glucose out of the lactic acid that has been building up within the muscle. If one looks at the biochemical equation for glycolysis one will note that it begins with glucose, and proceeds through several chemical conversions to glucose-6-phosphate, glucose 1,6-diphosphate, fructose-6-phosphate -- and proceeds until pyruvate is manufactured. This occurs in the cytosol, the outer liquid portion of the cell, and in the absence of oxygen, the end result of this process being the creation of 2 molecules and, as a side effect, a build up of pyruvate. Pyruvate is then shuttled into the mitochondria, where it goes through the Krebs Cycle to produce 36 additional ATP molecules that help continue to fuel the process of muscular contraction. A problem inherent in this cycling of enzymes is that the glycolysis cycle turns much quicker than the Krebs Cycle is able to process pyruvate. As a consequence, pyruvate begins to stack up and is acted upon by another enzyme, lactate dehydrogenase, which results in the production of lactate (lactic acid). Consequently, when a trainee is performing high-intensity muscular work, particularly with little respite in between his exercises, his muscles begin to stack up a large amount of lactate. This is occurring at the same time that the body is breaking glycogen down within the muscle to continue fueling the contraction process (a process known as glycogenolysis), which is occurring at a very rapid rate owing to the amplification cascade that attends mobilizing glycogen out of muscle during high-intensity activity. Consequently, the muscle quickly runs out of glucose in the process of generating so much lactate. This triggers a biological process into motion known as the Cori Cycle, in which the lactate that has been stacking up gets released from the cytosol into the general circulation. The lactate then moves through the general circulation into the central vein of the liver where it undergoes another biological process called gluconeogenesis, in which the lactate gets re-synthesized back into glucose for use in refueling the glycolysis cycle. The upshot of this complicated biochemical process is that when a trainee runs out of glycogen in his working muscles and his body liberates lactate into his bloodstream, his pH levels drop off markedly, producing a strong lactic acidosis and feelings of nausea. Such an occurrence can easily drop an individual's blood pH from 7.4 to 6.9, and when this happens, that is not an optimal pH for the proper functioning of all sorts of physiologic functions. [1] The muscle enzymes that produce the vascular tone in the smooth muscle of the blood vessels have a pKa of about 7.35, and when the pH level drops to 6.9, they simply can't function optimally. As a result, there is vasodilation, and one's blood pressure will drop to 80, and one will feel compelled to lie on the floor, overtaken by nausea, which is the natural result that attends inadequate blood flow to one's abdomen. These feelings can endure for 15 to 40-minutes, which is how long it takes for the circulating lactate to get to the central vein of the liver to undergo gluconeogenesis, the process that ups the glucose levels in the bloodstream and restores the blood sugar balance to the body. The question at this point then becomes: How can one workout in a high-intensity fashioin and not have this happen? The authors have found different solutions to this problem that are very effective. One method is pre-emptive, the other prescriptive. Given that such incidents occur almost exclusively in supervised workouts (largely because most people who are self-supervised won't push themselves hard enough to drain their muscles of glycogen to the degree necessary to engage the Cori Cycle), if the trainer is made aware of how the client is feeling, he can take steps to prevent the onset of such symptoms. This is accomplished by simply asking questions to the client as the workout proceeds in order to obtain feedback as to how he or she is feeling. If the client is starting to feel light-headed or nauseous, the trainer can choose to slow down the pace of the workout (by increasing the amount of time that the trainee takes in between exercises) so that the glycogen demands of the workout are not becoming urgent to his body. This gives his body more time to meet these demands, thus preventing the need for a lactate dump into the bloodstream. If, for instance, a trainee has been moving from one exercise station to the next in 15-seconds, if he doubles that time in between exercises to 30-seconds, this will allow his body 50 percent more time to keep pace with the energy demands.

> If someone is starting to feel light-headed during a workout, but tries to tough it out by proceeding with the workout at a quick pace, the sequential stacking of lactate will necessitate the lactate spilling into the central circulation so that it will be brought to the liver for the Cori Cycle - and then nausea occurs. So I try to not let it happen in the first place. Should it occur I think an appropriate recovery interval is very important because what's happening in that recovery interval is that you're actually allowing the Cori Cycle to function and therefore to up-regulate, which over time means that the client will develop a greater tolerance for the activity they are doing and won't become nauseated.
>
> **-- Doug McGuff, MD**

The prescriptive option has proven helpful to relieving the symptoms of light-headedness and nausea, and consists of merely administering sublingual sucrose (sugar under the tongue). Much like someone who might take Tylenol for pain relief, taking sugar prior to a workout or immediately upon the symptoms appearing, serves to remove these symptoms very quickly. The mechanism by which this works is pretty straight forward: It's in the nature of things that nausea or the feeling of nausea attends as a matter of course when the body, in an effort to keep one's muscles contracting will attempt to produce more glucose to help continue to fuel the contractions by either dumping the stacked up lactate into the bloodstream to trigger the Cori Cycle, which results in a lowering of one's pH levels and the nausea that goes with it. This process can be pre-empted, however, by taking sugar under the tongue, which staves off the need for the body to dump the lactate into the bloodstream. However, if we are constantly draining the glycogen out of the muscle/s, then we're always going to be one-step ahead of the process and the Cori Cycle is going to be tripped into motion and nausea will attend. The body, in other words, is always going to reach out to get whatever it can from the bloodstream to keep the wheels in motion for continued muscular contraction, and if sufficient glucose isn't there then the Cori Cycle is going to be engaged as a matter of course. It may not ever be something that you can dodge owing to the fact that it attends high order muscular effort. If someone does feel nauseous from working out, they can lie down with their feet elevated for upwards of 10 minutes or they can take sugar under their tongue – or they can do both. One can thus wait it out until one's system self-regulates its energy substrates, but this can take upwards of 30 minutes. In the meantime, the client is feeling terrible. Sugar administered sublingually will take away this feeling in as little as 30-seconds. Ideally, one should never get to the point where one is overtaken by feelings of light-headedness or nausea. And these feelings can be avoided altogether by either consuming some sugar immediately prior to the workout, during the workout or by backing off in how quickly one moves from station to station as one trains. These symptoms also tend to be more prominent with whole body workouts and often switching to a split routine will prevent such symptoms from occurring.

ARTHRITIS

QUESTION: I have arthritis. My question is do you think I can train with a Body By Science workout program and, if so, are there any precautions my trainer should take with me?

ANSWER: Selecting exercises that properly track

muscle and joint function is a built-in safety factor of the type of workout that we advocate. The "Big 5" exercises are fairly simple to perform and do not produce a lot of wear and tear on the joints and connective tissues and, thus, are comfortable for the joints involved in the exercises. If a trainee is arthritic, however, discomfort can attend the performance of these movements unless certain adjustments are made to the range of motion the arthritic joint is made to move through. For the trainee with arthritis we would recommend using the equipment in such a way as to delimit the range of motion so that the trainee is operating only within the comfortable range for that joint. However, the good news is that we've found that as the arthritic trainee's strength increases, he or she will be able to expand his or her range of motion in the "Big 5" workout over time. For instance on the Leg Press, we may only be able to have the trainee move his legs from full extension back to 45-degress to begin with, but within 6-to-12-weeks he'll be able to increase his hip flexion all the way back to 90-degrees because as he gradually becomes stronger his joints will become more tolerant of being moved through a full range of motion. A lot of what limits an arthritic joint's range of motion is not the derangement of the joint, per se, but rather the weakness of the surrounding supporting musculature outside joint angles that produce higher levels of force. For instance, when one's knee is fully extended and one has the bone-on-bone-tower, one can tolerate bearing a lot more weight, but as soon as the joint angle becomes more acute, then the force output from the muscle groups acting on that joint go down. The co-sign of 90-degrees is "0," so forced output as one approaches 90-degrees with one's elbow or hip joint is going to be lower. A weak person is not going to be able to tolerate approaching such joint angles, but as he becomes stronger the force output of his muscles is going to be greater, with the result that less advantageous joint angles are going to be better tolerated as his muscles will now be able to absorb that force and not transmit all of it to the joint. We have trained a lot of arthritic clients and we will typically start them out at a range of motion that seems to be a very short stroke, but as they get stronger, we will gap them out on the machine they are training on by a mere one hole or less every few weeks until they have achieved a full range of motion again –in spite of their arthritic joints. And as they continue to grow stronger, we will expand their range of motion at that same weight (we don't lower the weight as they increase their range) and they're able to tolerate it. Training in a limited range of motion has absolutely no negative consequences in so far as transferring to a full range of motion. It also speaks to the fact that a person with arthritis basically has a hinge that is rusty; and a rusty hinge can be moved through its full range of motion if there is enough capability to apply force for that hinge to operate at angles that transmit less force output. For instance, if you're doing a chest press, when your shoulder joint and your elbow joint approach 90-degrees, the amount of force being transmitted to the movement arm is minimum simply because the angle of pull on the shoulder joint is minimal. However, when a person is arthritic, all of that force is transmitted onto the joint and very little of that force will be absorbed by the muscle. The result being that the joint in question will not tolerate approaching that particular angle without pain. However, if the arthritic trainee can increase his strength by, say, 100 percent, the result is that his muscle will now be twice as strong and that force will now be absorbed into the muscle belly rather than being transmitted purely into the arthritic joint. As a consequence, the deranged joint can grow to tolerate being moved into its least advantageous position. Most elderly people that are stiff or prone to falls are not thusly afflicted because their joints are "stiff;" rather, they are suffering these infirmities owing to the fact that their musculature has grown so weak that they cannot tolerate coming out of a bone-on-bone-tower position.

COLDS

QUESTION: I'm a personal trainer and wanted to know if a client comes to your facility with a cold, do you think it's a good idea to train him?

ANSWER: If someone comes into one of our facilities with a cold and wants to workout we will typically send him home. A lot of what goes into our decision of course will depend upon the nature of the cold; i.e., if it's a minor cold, such that the client's throat simply feels a little scratchy but there's no fever (i.e., they're not febrile or feeling weak or have body ache), then we will typically allow him to workout. By contrast, if someone has a cold that's going to consume some of their adaptive energy, rather than having him perform a high-intensity workout that is going to mobilize amino acids out of the muscle and consume glutamine stores, he would be better served by resting to allow those amino acid and glutamine stores to be used as a backbone for anti-body synthesis (as opposed to trying to repair muscle tissue damage). The trainee must keep in mind that it takes adaptive resources to overcome a virus, so our inclination is that rather than workout, missing a workout is the trainee's chance to get over his cold and augment his recovery a little bit.

EQUIPMENT SAFETY

QUESTION: How important is regular equipment maintenance in the big picture of long-term safety and productive exercise? I mean, at the facility I workout at I never see anyone inspecting the equipment.

ANSWER: It's very important as sometimes injuries can occur at commercial facilities as a result of the proprietor not looking after his equipment. Take a moment to inspect the equipment you are going to be using (even if the proprietor doesn't) and make sure that nothing looks faulty. You wouldn't want to be performing Pulldowns with 210-pounds on the weight stack with a frayed cable. Make sure the equipment is safe, and that the guide rods are well lubricated and the movement arms move slowly and don't stick. Even from a training (rather than just a safety) standpoint this is important because you want to reach muscular failure, rather than being forced to stop due to a mechanical failure of the machine's movement arms. Other problems can occur depending upon what type of equipment one chooses in one's workouts. If, for instance, one elects to train with free weights, it would be wise to have a trainer or a training partner as free weights can be dangerous, particularly as the trainee fatigues and control is compromised.

TRAINING WHILE PREGNANT

QUESTION: I am a personal trainer and one of my clients recently told me that she was pregnant. I'm wondering if it is okay for me to train her during her pregnancy?

ANSWER: The type of training that we advocate in *Body By Science* is actually an ideal rehearsal for labor, which is characterized by intense muscular contractions with high metabolic demand and a high degree of exertional discomfort that one must breathe through without Val Salva. Consequently, there couldn't be a more perfect rehearsal for pregnant women to go through prior to labor. And one of the highest risks for non-progressive labor and the need for C-section is generally attributable to being in poor physical condition, which a proper training program will be very beneficial for remedying. As one progresses along in one's pregnancy and becomes larger, certain allowances must be made for the changes in a woman's body shape. As a woman's abdomen gets bigger, exercises such as prone Leg Curls will have to be omitted from her training. The lower turnaround portion of the Leg Press will also have to be adjusted. Exercises that require her to lie flat on her back will also have to excluded, as the uterus will compress the vena cava and inhibit blood return to the heart. Such minor adjustments to her workout will allow a woman who is pregnant to continue to workout very close to her delivery time. When she gets to within a few weeks of her delivery additional allowances will have to be made; she will need to reduce the amount of weight she is using in her workouts owing to the fact that the ligaments of her pelvis will start to soften as she starts to develop the ligamentous laxity in preparation for childbirth. But other than making certain allowances because of the physiology and body shape of pregnancy, it's desirable and safe to train through most of one's pregnancy. This is not to suggest that certain conditions that develop during pregnancy don't trump the workout, and these would be things a woman's OB should be able to tell her. Things such as conditions of Preeclampsia or hypertension in pregnancy, would be a reason to avoid working out; having a placental abruption or a separation of the placenta from the uterus (for whatever reason) would put a woman at strict bed rest without being able to workout; a placenta previa, where the placenta overlies the opening of the cervix is a reason not to workout; severe pregnancy related diabetes is a reason not to work out. So there are several things that would place a woman's pregnancy at high risk that would be good grounds to stop her from working out, but these would typically be communicated to the expectant mother by her OB. Apart from such considerations, and all other things being equal, a woman becoming stronger is definitely an asset for her going into labor. The most demanding athletic event the average female will ever go through in her life is childbirth. As such, if any athlete were going into the biggest athletic event of her life, you would think that she would want to train appropriately for that. And that is precisely what the kind of training that we advocate offers – the best training possible for the biggest athletic event of a woman's life. Such training also sets the woman up to have a quick recovery from her pregnancy because she will have bigger and stronger muscles, and one of the chief characteristics of muscle is tonus (the residual tension that exists within a muscle when it's not actively contracting). So if a woman is strong and she has a higher volume of muscle mass, then she is necessarily going to have a higher tonus. As a result, in terms of "snapping back," or regaining her pre-pregnancy shape, having a higher muscle mass, and, therefore, a greater tonus, will result in a quicker return to her pre-pregnancy shape. Now having said all this, you, as her trainer, must be especially cautious. As a rule of thumb, we advise female clients not to train during their first trimester, and it obviously isn't because we believe that the type of training that we advocate poses any risk or danger to her pregnancy, but rather because of the fact that roughly 25 percent of most pregnancies will have bleeding during the first trimester, and about one half of those will go on to miscarriage as a result of the fact that there is not enough genetic material present for the fetus to survive beyond this point. And as the natural human inclination is to try and blame someone or something for such a profound loss, if a trainee is working out at a personal training facility once a week, then that means that there is a one out of seven chance that should this event occur at all, it might occur on the same day as her workout -- and we don't think most training centers or trainers want to incur that risk.

SYMPTOMS TO WATCH FOR

QUESTION: Are there any symptoms I should be watching for when I workout – just to ensure that my health is not at risk?

ANSWER: Any type of physical training (including high-intensity training) carries some degree of risk. As to be "forewarned is to be forearmed," knowing what symptoms to look for can often prove helpful in preventing minor problems from becoming major ones. While we do tolerate a level of exertional discomfort that most people would consider abnormal and unpleasant during a workout, conditions such as the sudden onset of headache (or thunderclap headache), focal numbness or weakness in any part of the body, chest pain or chest pressure, unusual shortness of breath or any unusual degree of clamminess or sweatiness that are not context appropriate, would all be symptoms that should cause you to terminate your training and seek out competent medical attention.

HIGH INTENSITY TRAINING AND AORTIC DISSECTION

QUESTION: I've heard that there is a risk for aortic dissection with weight training. Even some trainers have said that this is true and have advised using techniques like Pre-Exhaust to limit the risk. Is this true?

ANSWER: Many of these trainers are misinformed and using Pre-Exhaust as a remedy to aortic dissection is simply incorrect because it's based on the assumption that strength training "causes" such a condition. The reality is that aortic dissection is a freak event that besets people that are predisposed to it as a result of a congenital connective tissue disorder. In other words, the fact that it beset them while they were working out with weights is simply a matter of "being on the bridge when lightning strikes." Were you to study the phenomenon of aortic dissections in general you would find a hundredfold more aortic dissections occurring when people are shopping or on the golf course, but no one's writing articles on the dangers of golfing or shopping and aortic dissection. Every once in a while, by sheer statistical fluke, you're going to have someone that dissects in and around the period that they have been lifting weights. But naturally everyone makes the jump backward to that as being what caused it. However, you must remember that *association* does not prove *causation*; after all, 90 percent of all people die in bed, but this doesn't prove that beds are dangerous. And to try and address it the way these trainers have done is to concede a premise that simply isn't correct.

COOLING DOWN AFTER EXERCISE

QUESTION: This is a short question that requires a long set up, so please bear with me. It's been reported that sudden death can occur not just during activity but after activities such as jogging or snow shoveling. When endurance exercise is stopped abruptly, the rate of electrical discharge by the pacemaker tissue of the heart decreases rapidly. Also, when aerobic exercise is performed in an upright position such as running or walking, blood tends to collect or pool in the lower half of the body. When exercise is stopped, the return of blood to the heart can sometimes be reduced, so that coronary blood flow falls below the level needed to provide appropriate oxygen to the heart. This can be aggravated by the "surge" of hormones adrenaline and noradrenaline that normally occurs in the immediate post-exercise period. As a result of this a spontaneous beat may be generated by muscle tissue in the heart ventricles (the main pumping chambers of the heart), especially when the coronary arteries supplying the heart are narrowed by arteriosclerosis. Such spontaneous ventricular beats are usually harmless but they can sometimes lead to ventricular fibrillation and sudden death. These difficulties – rapid decrease in heart rate, a pooling of blood in the lower body, and adrenaline surge – can be minimized by incorporating a minimum "cooling down period" of five to ten minutes after exercise. You don't address this in Body By Science, so I would like to ask what do you say to that?

ANSWER: "How?" is what we say to that. How does that help -- as opposed to just relaxing? Our argument would be that while that may be true, it's really an argument as to why strength training is superior. If you recall the study that we cited in Body By Science entitled Hemodynamic responses during leg press exercise in patients with chronic congestive heart failure by K. Meyer, et al., which was published in the. American Journal of Cardiology, 1999 Jun 1; 83(11): 1537-43, it clearly established that high-intensity strength training augments coronary return, which therefore augments coronary artery blood flow, and, thus, makes permissive a higher level of exertion without risk for coronary ischemia. And you're going to have enhanced coronary artery blood flow. What happens with low-intensity steady-state (aerobic) activity is that when you stop, there is has not been an intense enough muscular demand from this activity to augment venous return. So you have increased the myocardial oxygen demand in a context where you're not necessarily augmenting venous return. And particularly with jogging, where you might actually be pooling venous blood rather than returning it, this creates a mismatch of oxygen demand to coronary artery blood flow that can predispose you to arrhythmia. In Body By Science we also cited another study that examined a cardiac rehab program that incorporated both the traditional aerobic treadmill based cardiac rehab, along with high-intensity strength training and the incidence of arrhythmias in the strength training group was essentially "0," while there were arrhythmias and recurrent chest pains and other complications that were present in the treadmill based group. So the concept of needing a "cool down" period of steady-state activity (and we would also add the supposed "need" for a separate warm up period that includes activities such as stretching) is rendered obsolete by performing proper exercise.

NOTES ON TEXT

PART ONE:

1. Staron, RS et al. *Strength and skeletal muscle adaptations in heavy-resistance -trained women after detraining and retraining.* J Appi Physiol 1991 Feb; 70(2): 631-40.
2. Noakes, TD. Maximal oxygen uptake: "classical" versus "contemporary" viewpoints: a rebuttal. Med Sci Sports Exerc 1998 Sep;30(9): 1381-98. Noakes argues that the VO2max plateau occurs not because of central cardiovascular limitations, but because some central "governor" inhibits further skeletal muscle recruitment to protect the heart muscle from ischemia. This makes sense because the pumping capacity of the heart is both dependent on, but also a determinant of, its own blood supply. Thus exercise carried beyond the VO2 plateau will result in myocardial ischemia (which does not occur in the absence of coronary artery disease). Thus VO2max is a measure of, and limited by skeletal muscle factors, not central CV factors.
3. Saltin, B. et al. The nature of the training response; peripheral and central adaptations of one-legged exercise. Acta Physiol Scand. 1976 Mar; 96(3): 289-305.
4. Noakes, TD. Physiological models to understand exercise fatigue and the adaptations that predict or enhance athletic performance. Scand J Med Sci Sports 2000 Jun: 10(3): 123-45.
5. Page. 189, *The Paleolithic Prescription*, Perennial Library, Harper and Row, © 1988.

PART TWO:

1. Rader, Peary. The Rader Master Bodybuilding And Weight Gaining System, pg.36 © 1946, Ironman Publishing Co., Alliance, Nebraska. "It is not necessary, and is in fact unwise, to work out too often on this program ... and it is usually best to do but two workouts per week. Ansorge, one of the world's strongest men, worked out only once every

five days." Similarly, in a course pubished in 1941 by Bob Hoffman, we find the following: "While it is beneficial, after you are advanced, to work very hard one day a week...;" Bob Hoffman's Simplified System of Barbell Training © 1941 York Barbell Co., York, Pennsylvania.

2. Willoughby DS. Effects of an alleged myostatin-binding supplement and heavy resistance training on serum mysotatin, muscle strength and mass, and body composition. Int J Sport Nutr Exerc Metab. 2004 Aug; 14(4): 461-72.

PART THREE:

1. Kader DF, Wardlaw D, Smith FW; Correlation between the MRI Changes in the Lumbar Multifidus Muscles and Leg Pain. Clinical Radiology; February 2000 Volume 55, Number 2. Department of Radiology, Woodend Hospital. Aberdeen, United Kingdom. (Note: This study found multifidi muscle atrophy in 80% of patients with low back pain. Interestingly, clinical research using MedX to rehabilitate lumbar spine dysfunction boasts nearly an 80% success rate. Perhaps these figures are coincidentally similar. It is, however, tempting to speculate that the widespread multifidi muscle atrophy in this study and the targeted multifidi training afforded by MedX explain in part the widespread success of MedX therapy across diagnoses. That is, it is possible that various spinal pathologies share at least one common symptom generator: multifidi dysfunction. Thus, addressing this dysfunction should improve a majority of low back pain patients owing to their common trait of aberrant multifidi function. From these data, it can be argued that most patients with lumbar pain should receive physical therapy directed at reconditioning the multifidi.

2. Danneels LA, Vanderstraeten GG, Cambier DC, Witvrouw EE, De Cuyper HJ. CT Imaging of Trunk Muscles in Chronic Low Back Pain Patients and Healthy Control Subjects. European Spine Journal; August 2000 Volume 9, Number 4. Department of

Rehabilitation Sciences and Physical Therapy, Faculty of Medicine, Ghent University, Belgium. (Note: This research on nonoperative persons adds to the impressive body of evidence regarding a relationship between multifidi dysfunction and low back pain. It is not known if muscle weakness and atrophy are the cause or the result of chronic low back pain. It is possible that this relationship may depend upon the particular case. Weakness represents an abnormality that requires intervention in the form of isolated spinal strengthening to optimize spinal function.

3. Myer K and Hajric R, et.al. Hemodynamic responses during leg press exercise in patients with chronic congestive heart failure. *Am J Cardiol.* 1999 Jun 1; 83(11):1537-43.

4. Yeater R, Reed C, et. al. Resistance trained athletes using or not using steroids compared to runners: effects on cardiorespiratory variables, body composition and plasma lipids. *Br J Sports Med* 1996 Mar;30(1):11-4.

5. Degroot DW, et al. Circuit weight training in cardiac patients: determining optimal workloads for safety and energy expenditure. J Cardiopulm Rehabil. Mar-Apr;18(2):145-52._

6. Daub WD, et al. Strength training early after myocardial infarction. J Cardiopulm Rehabil. 1996 Mar-Apr;16(2):100-8._

7. Verrill DE, Ribisl PM. Resistive exercise training in cardiac rehabilitation. An update. *Sports Med* 1996 May;21(5):347-83.

8. Beniamini Y, et al. High-intensity strength training of patients enrolled in an outpatient cardiac rehabilitation program. J. Cardiopulm Rehabil 1999 Jan-Feb; 19(1):8-17.

9. Parker, ND et al. *Effects of strength training on cardiovascular responses during a submaximal walk and weight-loaded walking test in older females.* J. Cardiopulm Rehab 1996 Jan-Feb; 16(l):56-62.

10. Haykowsky MJ, et. al. Effects of long term resistance training on left ventricular morphology. *Can J Cardiol* 2000 Jan;16 (1):35-8.

11. McCartney N. Role of resistance training in heart

disease. *Med Sci Sports Exerc* 1988 Oct; 30(10 Suppl):S396-402.

12. McCartney N, et.al. Usefulness of weightlifting training in improving strength and maximal power output in coronary disease. *Am J Cardiol* 1991 May 1;67(11):939-45.

13. Stewart KJ. Resistive training effects on strength and cardiovascular endurance in cardiac and coronary prone patients. *Med Sci Sports Exerc* 1989 Dec;21(6):678-82.

14. Keleman MH, et. al. Circuit weight training in cardiac patients. *J Am Coll Cardiol* 1986 Jan;7(1):38-42.

15. Daub WD, et. al. Strength training early after myocardial infarction. *J Cardiopulm Rehabil* 1996 Mar-Apr;16(2):100-8.

16. McCartney N, McKelvie RS. The role of resistance training in patients with cardiac disease. *J Cardiovasc Risk* 1996 Apr;3(2):160-6.

17. Yamasaki H, et.al. Effects of weight training on muscle strength and exercise capacity in patients after myocardial infarction. *J Cardiol* 1995 Dec;26(6):341-7.

18. Stewart KJ, et. al .Safety and efficacy of weight training soon after acute myocardial infarction.. *J Cardiopulm Rehabil* 1998 Jan-Feb;18(1):37-44.

19. Martel GF, et. al. Strength training normalizes resting blood pressure in 65- to 73-year-old men and women with high normal blood pressure. *J Am Geriatr Soc* 1999 Oct;47(10):1215-21.

20. Kelley GA, Kelley KS. Progressive resistance exercise and resting blood pressure: A meta-analysis of randomized controlled trials. *Hypertension* 2000 Mar;35(3):838-43.

21. Harris KA, Holly RG. Physiological response to circuit weight training in borderline hypertensive subjects. *Med Sci Sports Exerc* 1987 Jun;19(3):246-52.

22. Blood pressure in resistance-trained athletes. Colliander EB, Tesch PA *Can J Sport Sci* 1988 Mar;13(1):31-4.

23. Sparling PB, et al. *Strength training in a cardiac rehabilitation program: a six-month follow-up.* Arch Phys Med Rehab 1990 Feb; 71(2).-148-52.

24. Hardy DO, Tucker LA. The effects of a single bout of strength training on ambulatory blood pressure levels in 24 mildly hypertensive men. Am J Health Promot 1998 Nov-Dec; 13(2):69-72. BP was monitored every 15mins after strength training for 24 hrs. "Systolic pressure and pressure load were reduced for at least 1 hour after exercise, and diastolic pressure and blood pressure load were reduced for 1 hour, 3 minutes after exercise."

25. Colliander EB, Tesch PA. Blood pressure in resistance-trained athletes. Can J Sport Sci 1988 Mar; 13(1):31-4. Conclusion: "Intense long-term strength training, as performed by bodybuilders, does not constitute a potential cardiovascular risk factor."

26. Dubach, P, et al. Effect of high intensity exercise training on central hemodynamic responses to exercise in men with reduced left ventricular function. J Am Coll Cadiol 1997 Jun; 29(7):1591-8. Showed improvements in VO2max and CO without worsening of hemodynamic status or further myocardial damage. Note: this was an interval protocol not weight training….but shows exertion is not dangerous.

PART FOUR:

1. H. S. Milner-Brown and colleagues. Journal of Physiology, 230, 359 (1973).
2. S. Grillner and M. Udo. Acta Pysiol. Scand., 81, 571 (1971).
3. H.S. Milner-Brown et al., J. Physiol., 230, 385 (1973).
4. Hutchins, Ken. *SuperSlow The ULTIMATE Exercise Protocol* Level I, Third Edition. Copyright 2007 SuperSlow Zone, LLC. Chapter 32, "The Ideal Exercise Environment" p 177-86.
5. Winning, losing, mood, and testosterone. McCaul, KD et al. Horm Behav. 1992 Dec; 26(4):486-504.
6. Effects of ability-and chance-determined competition outcome on testosterone. Van Anders, SM, Watson, NV. Physiol Behav. 2007 Mar 16; 90 (4): 634-42. Epub 2007 Jan 16.

7. Testosterone change after losing predicts the decision to compete again. Mehta PH, Josephs RA. Horm Behav. 2006 Dec; 50(5):684-92. Epub 2006 Aug 22.
8. Testosterone changes during vicarious experiences of winning and losing among fans at sporting events. Bernhardt PC, et al. Physiol Behav. 1998 Aug; 65(1): 59-62.

PART FIVE:

1. Cordain, L. et al. The Paradoxical nature of hunter-gatherer diets: meat-based, yet non-atherogenic. Eur J Clin Nutr. 2002 Mar; 56 Suppl: S42-52.
2. O'Keefe JH Jr, Cordain L. Cardiovascular disease resulting from a diet and lifestyle at odds with our Paleolithic genome: how to become a 21st-century hunter-gatherer. Mayo Clin Proc. 2004 Jan; 79(1): 101-8
3. Cordain L. et al. Plant-animal subsistence ratios and macronutrient energy estimations in worldwide hunter-gatherer diets. Am J Clin Nutr. 2000 Mar; 71(3):682-92. *This demonstrates high reliance on animal based foods and relatively low carbohydrate content, with carbs consumed from low carb plant food sources.*
4. Collins, C. Said another way: stroke, evolution and the rainforests: an ancient approach to modern healthcare. Nurs Forum. 2007 Jan-Mar; 42(1): 39-44. *"The race is on, therefore, to learn what we can about diet, exercise, and natural medicine from the last few humans who live lifestyles that might be closest to our natural state.*
5. O'Dea K. Cardiovascular disease risk factors in Australian aborigines. Clin Exp Pharmacol Physiol. 1991 Feb; 18(2): 85-8. ..."*a diet of low energy density and high nutrient density derived from very lean wild meat, and uncultivated vegetable foods. It has important therapeutic implications for the treatment and prevention of many of the chronic degenerative diseases of affluent Western societies.*

6. Simopoulos AP, Evolutionary aspects of omega-3 fatty acids in the food supply. Prostaglandins Leukot Essent Fatty Acids. 1999 May-Jun; 60(5-6):421-9.
7. Simopouls AP. Evolutionary aspects of diet, the omega-6/omega-3 ratio and genetic variation: nutritional implications for chronic diseases. Biomed Pharmcother. 2006 Nov; 60(9): 502-7.
8. Simopoulos AP. Human requirements for N-3 polyunsaturated fatty acids. Poult Sci. 2000 Jul; 79(7):961-70.
9. Lemon, Peter, PhD, International Journal of Sport Nutrition, 1998; 8; 426-447.

PART SIX:

1. Kelly, Friery, Bishop, Phillip. Long-Term Impact Of Athletic Participation On Physical Capabilities. Journal of Exercise Physiologyonline (JEPonline). Volume 10 Number 1 February 2007.
2. Children's Hospital Boston web page: http://www.childrenshospital.org/az/Site1112/printerf riendlypageS1112P0.html
3. SafeKidsUSA website: http://www.usa.safekids.org/tier3_cd.cfm?folder_id= 540&content_item_id=1211
4. Some of the studies reviewed in his research included: Brown, E.W., and RS. Kimball. Medical history associated with adolescent powerlifting. *Pediatrics72:636*-644.1983; Kristiansen, B. Association football injuries in schoolboys. *Scand.J. Sports Sci.* 5(1):1-2.1983; McCracken, P. Will rugby scar your child for life? *Personality Magazine* (South Africa). pp. 18-20. May 1989; Ryan, J.R, and G.G. Salciccioli. Fractures of the distal radial epiphyses in adolescent weightlifters. *Am. J.Sports;* Sparks, J.P. Half a million hours of Rugby football. Br.*J. Sports Med.* 15:30-32.1981; Zaricznyj, B.,L.J.M.Shattuck, T.A. Mast, RV. Robertson and G. D'Elias. Sports related injuries in school aged children.*Am.J.Sports.*
5. Hamill, B.P.Relative safety of weightlifting and weight training. *J. Strength and CondoRes.* 8(1):53-57.1994.

6. Schmidtbleicher, D. An interview on strength training for children. *Nat. Strength CondoAssoc. Bulletin* 9(12):42a-42b.198820).

7. Ericsson, K.A., Krampe, R. T.H., Tesch-Romer, The Role of Deliberate Practice In the Acquisition of Expert Performance. Psychological Review (1993), 100 (3), pgs 379-384.

8. Medicine & Science in Sports & Exercise. 36(3):371-378, March 2004; *The Impact of Stretching on Sports Injury Risk: A Systematic Review of the Literature; THACKER, STEPHEN B. 1; GILCHRIST, JULIE 2; STROUP, DONNA F. 3; KIMSEY, C. DEXTER JR. 3.*

9. "New Study Links Stretching with Higher Injury Rates," Running Research News, Vol. 10(3), pp. 5-6, 1994.

10. *B M J* 2002;325:468 (31 August); *Effects of stretching before and after exercising on muscle soreness and risk of injury: systematic review;* Rob D Herbert, *senior lecturer,* Michael Gabriel, *physiotherapist.* School of Physiotherapy, University of Sydney, PO Box 170, Lidcombe, New South Wales 1825, Australia.

11. *Medicine & Science in Sports & Exercise* 2000;32:271–7. Pope RP, Herbert RD, Kirwan JD, et al. A randomized trial of preexercise stretching for prevention of lower-limb injury.

12. Witvrouw, E., Et al. (2007). *The role of stretching in tendon injuries.* Br J Sports Med. 41:226-226.

13. http://saveyourself.ca/bibliography.php?her00

14. Medicine & Science in Sports & Exercise: Volume 38(5) Supplement, May 2006p S294; *A Single Thirty Second Stretch Is Sufficient to Inhibit Maximal Voluntary Strength:* Nelson, Arnold G. FACSM; Winchester, Jason B, Kokkonen; Joke (LSU, Baton Rouge, LA; BYU-Hawaii, Laie, HI.)

ABOUT THE AUTHORS

Both Dr. Doug McGuff and John Little are owners of personal training centers, where, for over 12 years they have been training people on a one-to-one basis within the spirit (if not the letter) of scientific law. Moreover, they are both highly sought after consultants by athletes, bodybuilders, and all of those who desire maximum results in minimum time. Their individual books on exercise are best sellers and both conduct successful consultation businesses. Having supervised in excess of 150,000 one-on-one workouts between them, they are preeminently qualified to write THE authoritative text on training to achieve total fitness.

Doug McGuff MD is a partner with Blue Ridge Emergency Physicians, P.A. and the proprietor of Ultimate-Exercise, a state-of-the-art personal training facility in Seneca, South Carolina (www.ultimate-exercise.com). He is the author of *Ultimate-Exercise* and *BMX Training: A Scientific Approach*. Dr. McGuff lectures on exercise science all over the world.

John Little is, in *Ironman* magazine's words, "one of the leading fitness researchers in North America." He and his wife Terri own and operate Nautilus North: Strength & Fitness Centre, (www.nautilusnorth.com). He is the author of over 40 titles, ranging from history and philosophy to martial arts and strength fitness. His books *Max Contraction Training* and *Advanced Max Contraction Training* are considered classics in the strength fitness industry. (www.maxcontraction.com).